RECENT ADVANCES IN HEMATOLOGY RESEARCH

ANEMIA

PREVALENCE, RISK FACTORS AND MANAGEMENT STRATEGIES

RECENT ADVANCES IN HEMATOLOGY RESEARCH

Additional books in this series can be found on Nova's website under the Series tab.

Additional e-books in this series can be found on Nova's website under the e-book tab.

RECENT ADVANCES IN HEMATOLOGY RESEARCH

ANEMIA

PREVALENCE, RISK FACTORS AND MANAGEMENT STRATEGIES

ALICE HALLMAN
EDITOR

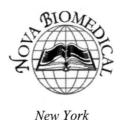

New York

Copyright © 2014 by Nova Science Publishers, Inc.

All rights reserved. No part of this book may be reproduced, stored in a retrieval system or transmitted in any form or by any means: electronic, electrostatic, magnetic, tape, mechanical photocopying, recording or otherwise without the written permission of the Publisher.

For permission to use material from this book please contact us:
Telephone 631-231-7269; Fax 631-231-8175
Web Site: http://www.novapublishers.com

NOTICE TO THE READER

The Publisher has taken reasonable care in the preparation of this book, but makes no expressed or implied warranty of any kind and assumes no responsibility for any errors or omissions. No liability is assumed for incidental or consequential damages in connection with or arising out of information contained in this book. The Publisher shall not be liable for any special, consequential, or exemplary damages resulting, in whole or in part, from the readers' use of, or reliance upon, this material. Any parts of this book based on government reports are so indicated and copyright is claimed for those parts to the extent applicable to compilations of such works.

Independent verification should be sought for any data, advice or recommendations contained in this book. In addition, no responsibility is assumed by the publisher for any injury and/or damage to persons or property arising from any methods, products, instructions, ideas or otherwise contained in this publication.

This publication is designed to provide accurate and authoritative information with regard to the subject matter covered herein. It is sold with the clear understanding that the Publisher is not engaged in rendering legal or any other professional services. If legal or any other expert assistance is required, the services of a competent person should be sought. FROM A DECLARATION OF PARTICIPANTS JOINTLY ADOPTED BY A COMMITTEE OF THE AMERICAN BAR ASSOCIATION AND A COMMITTEE OF PUBLISHERS.

Additional color graphics may be available in the e-book version of this book.

Library of Congress Cataloging-in-Publication Data

ISBN: 978-1-63321-775-1

Published by Nova Science Publishers, Inc. † New York

Contents

Preface		vii
Chapter 1	Anemia in Heart Diseases *Estelle Torbey, M.D. and Gretta Torbey, M.D.*	1
Chapter 2	Influence of Iron Deficiency Anaemia and Recovery on Oxidative/Antioxidant Status *Javier Díaz-Castro, Mario Pulido-Moran, Silvia Hijano, Naroa Kajarabille and Julio J. Ochoa*	19
Chapter 3	Influence of Iron Deficiency Anaemia on Bone Metabolism *Javier Díaz-Castro, Silvia Hijano, Mario Pulido-Moran, Naroa Kajarabille and Julio J. Ochoa*	35
Chapter 4	Sickle Cell Anemia: Prevalence, Risk Factors and Management Strategies *Bruna Miglioranza Scavuzzi, Lucia Helena da Silva Miglioranza and Isaias Dichi*	49
Chapter 5	Anemia in Myelodysplastic Syndromes *Alicia Enrico, M.D., María Gabriela Flores, M.D., Laura Kornblihtt, M.D., Ph.D., Elsa Nucifora, M.D., Yesica Bestach, M.Sc., Irene B. Larripa, Ph.D., and Carolina B. Belli, Ph.D.*	65

Chapter 6	Transfusion in Chronic Anaemia *Philip Crispin*	99
Chapter 7	Anaemia: Prevalence, Risk Factors and Management with a Focus on Chronic Kidney Disease *K. Abdul Razak, D.W. Mudge and D. W. Johnson*	123
Chapter 8	Strategy for Treating Anemia in Chronic Kidney Disease Patients from the Standpoint of Iron Utility *Daisuke Harada, Takehisa Kawata and Masaaki Inaba*	147
Chapter 9	Parasitic Anemia: Prevalence, Risk and Management *Somsri Wiwanitkit and Viroj Wiwanitkit*	165
Index		171

Preface

This book begins by discussing the effects anemia has on heart diseases. The book then continues to discuss the influence of iron deficiency anemia and recovery on oxidative/antioxidant status; influence of iron deficiency anemia on bone metabolism; sickle cell anemia; anemia in myelodysplastic syndromes; transfusion in chronic anemia; the prevalence, risk factors and management with a focus on chronic kidney disease; strategy for treating anemia in chronic kidney disease patients from the standpoint of iron utility; and parasitic anemia.

Chapter 1 – Anemia is defined as the decrease in the hemoglobin from normal values either by loss of red blood cells or deficit in production or both. Hemoglobin is the major transporter of oxygen. The variation in hemoglobin is therefore a factor in determining the cardiac output. Consequently anemia has important consequences on the normally functioning heart as well as the diseased heart including the ischemic and the failing heart Anemia is also a prognostic factor of several heart conditions. It is one of the determinants of the functional capacity in these conditions as well as survival. Furthermore, the treatment of anemia has its effect on the heart through variable mechanisms. On the other hand, the pathogenesis of anemia in heart diseases is multifactorial. The decrease in erythropoietin production, inflammatory cytokines secretion as well as concomitant iron deficiency and kidney diseases all contribute the occurrence of anemia in heart diseases. Consequently anemia worsens the underlying heart disease and at the same time is perpetuated by the cardiac condition. This closed cycle makes the pathophysiology and the treatment of either condition very intricate and will be discussed in detail in this chapter.

Chapter 2 – Oxidative stress results from an imbalance between the formation and neutralization of ROS and it is imposed on cells as a result of one or more of the following factors: an increase in oxidant generation, a decrease in antioxidant protection, or a failure to repair oxidative damage. There is controversy about the susceptibility of cells to lipid peroxidation in Fe deficiency anaemia: some investigators have claimed there is no difference in lipid peroxidation among patients with Fe deficiency anaemia compared with controls, but others have reported that among patients with IDA oxidants are increased and antioxidants decreased, so the oxidative/antioxidative balance is shifted toward the oxidative side. This apparent discrepancy may be due to different concentrations of ROS and antioxidant enzymes in the tissues studied, the subjects of the study, the severity of the Fe-deficiency and the methods used for the assessment of the oxidative stress. However, in humans, were the degree of Fe-deficiency is not very high, it is accepted that Fe-deficiency increases oxidative stress, fact that can also be attributed to the repletion process with several sources of Fe. Several authors have reported increased lipid peroxidation products in patients with Fe deficiency anaemia, which may be attributed to over production of ROS and a deficiency of antioxidant defense. Decreased SOD activity in Fe deficiency anaemia may be linked to increased oxidative stress, because it is well known that ROS, inhibit SOD activity. Other authors also found that CAT activity was significantly decreased in Fe-deficiency groups as compared with controls. CAT is an iron-dependent enzyme and is not unexpected to be decreased in iron deficiency.

Chapter 3 – There is a growing body of evidence from animal research, epidemiologic, and clinical studies indicating an association between osteopenia and anaemia. Fe intake is directly correlated with mineral bone density and Fe deficiency diminishes the mineral bone content, the bone mass and mechanical resistance. There is also an association of hemoglobin levels with the cortical bone mineralization and density. Several diseases characterized by low hemoglobin levels or Fe deficiency anemia have been associated with an increased risk of bone loss or osteoporosis. In fact, pernicious anemia is directly correlated with increased risk of osteoporotic fractures. Fe deficieny diminishes bone matrix formation, reducing the amount of procollagen type I N-terminal propeptide released to the sreum under these conditions.

Bone resorption process increases in Fe deficiency as shown by the increase of serum parathyroid hormone, tartrate-resistant acid phosphatase and levels of degradation products from C-terminal telopeptides of type I collagen. In addition, mineralization process is also affected by Fe deficiency, because

Ca and P content in femur decreases markedly, due to the increase in PTH and cortisol induced by Fe deficiency. Osteoblast function and bone formation are strongly oxygen-dependent. Hypoxic condition (a consequence from decreased oxygen delivery in Fe deficiency anaemia) diminishes bone formation. The inhibitory effects of hypoxia are due to decreased osteoblast proliferation and differentiation. In addition, hypoxia stimulate osteoclast activity in favor of pathological resorption. In conclusion, Fe deficiency anaemia has a significant impact upon bone, affecting bone mineralization, decreasing the matrix formation and increasing bone resorption, therefore it is of great interest to assess bone status in situation of Fe deficiency anaemia.

Chapter 4 – Sickle cell anemia (SCA) is a chronic illness and is one of the most common severe monogenic disorders in the world. Organ damage, brain dysfunction and the painful vaso-occlusive crises are serious complications affecting individuals with this disease. It is mostly common among people whose ancestors emigrated from Sub-Saharan Africa, South America, Cuba, Central America, Saudi Arabia, India, and Mediterranean countries such as Turkey, Greece, and Italy. The disease affects millions of people around the world and occurs in about one in every 500 African-American births and one in every 1000 to 1400 Hispanic-American births. In many cases, SCA is usually diagnosed with newborn screening. Vaccines, antibiotics, and folic acid supplements are administered, in addition to analgesics. Blood transfusions are a common management strategy, and the only known cure at present is by bone marrow transplant. This work discusses the pathophysiological process, the pharmaceutical and nutritional interventions used as well as specific complications management. Stem-cell transplantation techniques and gene therapy are mentioned. The drugs evaluated in-vitro, and some promising pharmaceuticals are also approached in this review.

Chapter 5 – One of the most challenging problems in hematology is the heterogeneous group of disorders that were formally defined as Myelodysplastic Syndromes (MDS) by the French–American–British Cooperative Group in 1982. MDS are clonal disorders of hematopoietic stem cells with a propensity to leukemic evolution. Idiopathic MDS occur mainly in older persons with an incidence of 5 per 100,000 persons per year in the general population that increases to 20 to 50 per year after 60 years of age.

The bone marrow is normo/hiper-cellular, displays various morphologic abnormalities and the stem cells show defective capacity for self-renewal and differentiation leading into an ineffective hematopoiesis. Most patients are initially asymptomatic, and their condition is incidentally discovered on a routine blood test.

Approximately 80% of patients manifest with anemia at diagnosis, and this percentage is increased in parallel with the evolution of the disease, being one of the hallmarks. The anemia is frequently macrocytic but refractory to treatment with folate and vitamin B12.

The clinical course of MDS is highly variable, ranging from stable disease over 10 years to death within a few months due to complications associated with their cytopenias or leukemic transformation. Since the development of the Bournemouth index in 1985, various scoring systems have been designed, based on clinical characteristic at presentation, in order to define prognostic subgroups. Anemia is well established as a negative prognostic factor. The International Prognostic Scoring System, the gold standard for risk assessment, has been recently revised (IPSS-R) where new clinical relevant cut-points for hemoglobin level were defined, among other changes. In our series of 578 (324 patients belong to the Argentinean MDS Registry) *de novo* MDS patients, the degree of anemia shows a good reproducibility and effectiveness to predict clinical outcome. Patients were distributed according to the IPSS-R cut-points for hemoglobin level into: 256 (44%) ≥10 g/dL, 191 (33%) 8-9.9 g/dL and 131 (23%) <8 g/dL, with median survival of 60, 35, and 19 months, and time to leukemic evolution (25% of patients) of 66, 23 and 14 months, respectively (p<0.001).

The relationship between severe anemia and poor clinical outcome suggests that anemia initiates or exacerbates functional decline, particularly, involving cardiovascular disease which is one of the most common co-morbidity in MDS patients. Also, there is a high prevalence of patients with transfusion dependence who are prompt to develop secondary iron overload, associated with clinical organ dysfunction, increased risk of cardiac failure, and reduced survival.

The great variability in the outcome of MDS complicates decision-making regarding therapies and prognostic characterization of individual patients is vital prior initiating treatment. The main objective in lower risk patients is improving the quality of life, and in higher risk patients is to extend the survival trying to modify the natural history of the disease. Accordingly, therapies vary from supportive care to intensive chemotherapy and stem cell transplantation.

The degree of anemia is one of the major criteria for diagnosis, prognosis and to proper select type and timing of treatment in MDS patients.

Chapter 6 – For the practicing haematologist, one of the most common transfusion decisions is in the chronically anaemic patient. There are unique aspects to this decision in sickle cell disease, where a body of evidence has developed around preventing complications of the underlying disease. In children, where chronic anaemia may lead to developmental concerns, transfusion goals may be formulated to prevent long term complications. In adults, chronic anaemia is most frequently seen in haematological malignancies and myelodysplasia, with the prevalence increasing with age. Transfusion decisions are therefore complicated by comorbid conditions of aging, such as cardiovascular and respiratory illness.

There is consensus in many published guidelines that transfusion is usually appropriate when the haemoglobin is less than 60-70g/L, and generally not indicated when the haemoglobin is more than 100g/L. This is despite evidence that there is a continuum of improvement in quality of life as the haemoglobin increases above these levels with the use of erythropoietin in myelodysplasia, cancer therapy and renal disease. Even with haemoglobins within the normal range, performance in trained athletes improves as the haemoglobin rises, either induced by erythropoietin or transfusion.

Patients usually are not aiming to achieve the levels of performance required in athletes. They may well cope with lower haemoglobin levels, and the weight of opinion supports this. However, there are no good laboratory measures to indicate when a low haemoglobin might be impairing function and considerable variability in practice, suggesting that the management of chronically anaemic patients is not optimal. This review will summarise the evidence guiding transfusion for relief of symptoms of anaemia in the chronic setting.

Chapter 7 – The global prevalence of anaemia has decreased over the last 20 years from 40.2% in 1990 to 32.9% in 2010, but with a significant geographical variation. Iron deficiency, the commonest cause, decreased as a proportion, whereas the anaemia of chronic kidney disease increased. Anaemia due to haemoglobinopathies remained relatively constant. The increasing anaemia in kidney disease coupled with ageing and population growth resulted in a dramatic increase in the number of patients in this group. Higher income regions have a higher proportion of haemoglobinopathies, kidney disease and gastrointestinal bleeding. Among the elderly, nutrition, kidney disease and its other associated risk factors (diabetes mellitus, hypertension and cardiovascular disease) were the greatest contributors to anaemia. The focus of this article is iron deficiency anaemia related to kidney disease, its risk factors and management strategies. Iron supplementation remains the cornerstone treatment of iron deficiency and the anaemia of kidney disease. Early and correct diagnosis of iron deficiency along with optimisation of iron stores is also the primary aim of the management of the cardiorenal syndrome and anaemia in diabetes. Recent trials comparing various oral iron formulations have yielded conflicting results. Newer intravenous preparations including ferric carboxymaltose and ferumoxytol have simplified management by permitting safer high-dose administration. Erythropoietin stimulating agents are also established therapy for patients with anaemia and kidney disease, and are used in early kidney disease, diabetes and the cardiorenal syndrome. However recent large trials have raised concern over the safety of these agents in treating anaemia, particularly at high doses.

Chapter 8 – Anemia is a common complication in patients with chronic kidney disease (CKD). In the past, clinical evidence has accumulated indicating that anemia is associated with higher mortality in CKD patients. Although erythropoiesis-stimulating agents (ESAs) had been considered to contribute to an improved quality of life in CKD patients, recent randomized controlled trials elucidated that high target hemoglobin levels in patients receiving ESAs were associated with an increased risk of cardiovascular events and death, due partly to either erythropoietin resistance or to preexisting cardiovascular disease (CVD). There are many factors associated with erythropoietin resistance, and inefficient iron utilization has been considered to be one of the main factors. For patients with erythropoietin resistance, it is necessary to increase the dose of intravenous (IV) iron to maintain appropriate levels of transferrin saturation (TSAT). However, excess iron use is followed by resultant increases in either serum ferritin or hepcidin, which are known to be independent factors associated with increased mortality in dialysis patients. Accumulating evidence, including that from the Dialysis Outcomes and Practice Patterns Study, has indicated that a reduction of the IV iron dose by itself, along with the resultant reduction of the serum ferritin or hepcidin levels, might improve the mortality in dialysis patients. Dialysis therapy in Japan has met with greater success than that other countries in terms of the improvement of mortality.

The authors have recently reported that a long-acting ESA, darbepoetin (DPO)-α, had more potent suppressive effects on the serum hepcidin level than short-acting erythropoietin, and that the serum ferritin level and the dose of IV iron were reduced in the patients on DPO-α to maintain the Hb and TSAT. This data clearly indicate that DPO-α is superior to ESA with regard to improving the iron utility, and thus the life expectancy, in dialysis patients.

Chapter 9 – Anemia is a common hematological problem that can be seen worldwide and it is still under consideration for global public health. There are many causes of anemia.

An important cause is the parasitic infestation. The parasitic anemia can be seen worldwide and this is still the problem in many countries, especially for those in tropical zone. There are many parasites that can induce anemia. In this short article, the authors will summarize and discuss on important kinds of parasitic anemia focusing on prevalence, risk and management.

In: Anemia
Editor: Alice Hallman

ISBN: 978-1-63321-775-1
© 2014 Nova Science Publishers, Inc.

Chapter 1

Anemia in Heart Diseases

Estelle Torbey[1],, M.D., and Gretta Torbey[2], M.D.*
[1]Staten Island University Hospital, New York, US
[2]Cochin Hospital, Paris, France

Abstract

Anemia is defined as the decrease in the hemoglobin from normal values either by loss of red blood cells or deficit in production or both. Hemoglobin is the major transporter of oxygen. The variation in hemoglobin is therefore a factor in determining the cardiac output. Consequently anemia has important consequences on the normally functioning heart as well as the diseased heart including the ischemic and the failing heart Anemia is also a prognostic factor of several heart conditions. It is one of the determinants of the functional capacity in these conditions as well as survival. Furthermore, the treatment of anemia has its effect on the heart through variable mechanisms. On the other hand, the pathogenesis of anemia in heart diseases is multifactorial. The decrease in erythropoietin production, inflammatory cytokines secretion as well as concomitant iron deficiency and kidney diseases all contribute the occurrence of anemia in heart diseases. Consequently anemia worsens the underlying heart disease and at the same time is perpetuated by the cardiac condition. This closed cycle makes the pathophysiology and the

---

* Corresponding author: Estelle Torbey, Heart Tower, Department of Cardiology, 475 Seaview Avenue, New York, NY. Email: Estelle_t83@hotmail.com.

treatment of either condition very intricate and will be discussed in detail in this chapter.

Introduction

The coexistence of anemia and heart disease is common. Patients with heart disease who are anemic have worse outcome then those with normal hemoglobin. While the exact etiology of anemia in that specific patient population remains unknown, the pathogenesis is multifactorial and complex. This chapter reviews the pathophysiology and treatment of anemia in heart failure as well as in acute and chronic artery disease.

Definition and Manifestations

Anemia is defined by the World Health Organization as hemoglobin <12 g/dl in women and <13 g/dl in men. Severe anemia is defined as hemoglobin <9g/dl. The prevalence of anemia in patients with heart failure varies from 22% to 46% [1] while its occurrence varies between 10 and 20% in those with chronic coronary artery disease [2]. Women and elderly with heart disease tend to have the highest prevalence of anemia [3].

Anemic patients develop several cardiac manifestations such as tachyarrhythmia (mostly sinus tachycardia and ectopy), exertional dyspnea, worsening of chronic coronary artery disease symptoms and dizziness but rarely syncope. Anemia can also cause acute chest pain and acute pulmonary edema either due to anemia itself or following transfusion. Patients with severe anemia also tend to have a systolic soft murmur.

Pathophysiology of Anemia in Heart Disease

Although the pathogenesis of anemia in heart disease is not fully delineated, several factors are believed to contribute to the development of anemia in this setting.

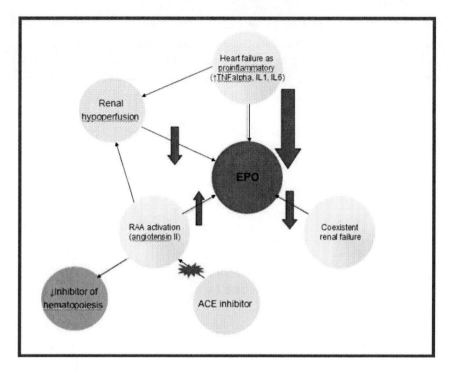

Figure 1. Pathophysiology of Anemia in Heart Failure. Role of erythropoietin. The decrease in erythropoietin level is due to renal hypoperfusion, administration of ACE inhibitors and proinflammatory agents that are secreted in the setting of heart failure. ACE =Angiotensin Convertase Inhibitor; EPO=Erythropoietin ;TNF=Tumor Necrosis Factor.

Heart Failure

Heart failure is an inflammatory state. In that setting, anemia is mainly due to both a decreased level of erythropeitin (EPO) (Figure 1) and to a state of iron deficiency.

The pro-inflammatory cytokines such as tumor necrosis factor alpha, interleukins 1 and 6 are believed to reduce (EPO) production and to induce resistance to its actions on the bone marrow [4-5]. The activated renin-angiotensin-aldosterone and sympathetic nervous systems in heart failure lead to renal hypoperfusion causing increased EPO production [6]. Angiotensin II increases directly EPO production and catabolizes inhibitors of hematopoiesis [7]. This increase is counterbalanced by a decrease in EPO due to the activity of cytokines, the usual coexistent renal dysfunction as well as the blocking activity of heart failure medications such as ACE inhibitors. EPO has also a range of cardiovascular effects. Its role encompasses myocardial protection and angiogenesis, activation of platelets and up-regulation of plasminogen activator inhibitor-1 [8]. This interaction of anemia, heart disease and kidney disease led to the definition of the cardio-renal syndrome as a "state in which therapy to relieve congestive HF symptoms is limited by further worsening kidney function" [9] and the cardiorenal anemia syndrome where anemia can be the cause or consequence of heart failure and chronic kidney disease [10]. In the setting of acute coronary syndrome, the exact contribution of EPO versus anemia itself in acute coronary syndrome (ACS) is not known.

Acute Coronary Syndrome

The decreased erythropoeisis in heart failure is not only due to EPO deficiency but also to the concomitant existing iron deficiency state. (Figure 2).

Iron deficiency in heart failure is thought to result from cardiac cachexia, poor intestinal absorption, gastrointestinal bleed when on chronic antiplatelets and impaired iron metabolism despite normal iron stores. In patients with ACS, iron deficiency seems to result from bleeding. Among those patients who are on aspirin, clopidogrel or prasugrel, 4% develop serious bleeding (intracranial or not, spontaneous or instrumentation-induced) [11]. In this setting, mortality following bleeding is initially high with a hazard ratio of 5.84 (95% CI 4.11-8.29) in the first day then mortality drops sharply over time. The risk resolves after 40 days. [11] In patients who undergo fibrinolytic and antithrombin therapies for STEMI, cardiogenic shock, age and intracranial hemorrhage are important independent indicators of 30-day and 1-year mortality, while in-hospital non-intracranial hemorrhage major and minor bleeding have no significant association with mortality. Patients who are older, female, non-smoker, who have lower body weight, who have higher TIMI risk score, who had a GPIIb/IIIa inhibitor are also more likely to develop bleeding in such a setting. Serious bleeding is more common with prasugrel than with clopidogrel [11-12]. In all these studies, the impact of bleeding on mortality is to be carefully considered since bleeding is a post-randomization event, therefore allowing for confounding factors to interfere with analysis.

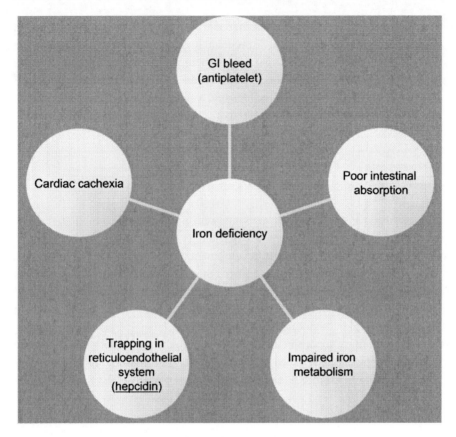

Figure 2. Pathophysiology of Anemia in Heart Failure: Role of Iron Deficiency. Iron deficiency affects heart failure at several stages:absorption, production and availability of iron to red blood cells and tissues. GI= Gastrointestinal.

Iron deficiency can result also from intrareticular retention. Hepcidin, a small peptide produced by the liver is thought to play an important role in trapping iron in the reiculoendothelial system and preventing the release of iron from the liver cells as well as the uptake of dietary iron by the gut mucosa [13-14].

Pregnancy

Anemia occurs also in the setting of pregnancy as a result of an increase in plasma volume that is more extensive than the increase in red blood cell count. The resulting relative anemia leads to a 20% raise in the heart rate which increases the cardiac output. This increase is well tolerated by women with normal hearts but not by the 2% pregnant women who have cardiovascular diseases. Neither those with impaired ventricular function and limited cardiac reserve nor those with left heart obstruction such as mitral stenosis, left ventricular outflow obstruction or bicuspid valve stenosis and regurgitation [15] tolerate anemia in pregnancy and have a high rate of maternal and fetal mortality.

Prosthetic Devices

Hemolysis is the culprit in patients with paraprosthetic valvular leakage and in those with assisted ventricular devices either due to the intrinsic continuous impella flow or to the development of thrombus [17].

Gastrointestinal bleeding is another common cause of anemia in patients with coronary artery disease on chronic antiplatelets or patient with atrial fibrillation on anticoagulants as well as patients with heart failure with an assisted ventricular device in place [18]. In the latter subgroup of patients, bleeding is thought to originate from an acquired von Willebrand syndrome due to shear stress and reduced pulsatility of the new continuous flow assisted device resulting in an increase in the prevalence of atriovenous malformations [19].

Effects of Anemia on Heart Disease

Anemia can result from defective erythropoiesis or excessive blood loss as previously described. It results in decreased oxygen delivery to tissues such as the myocardium in the territories of coronary stenosis [20]. To ensure adequate systemic oxygen delivery, a higher cardiac output is necessary, leading to increased stroke volume and heart rate and hence cardiac oxygen consumption [21]. The acute cardiac response consists of an increase in the cardiac output to compensate for hypoxemia and tissue hypoxia. This is ensured by both rapid heart rate and rapid velocity flow. Subsequently myocardial oxygen demand and consumption increase, which worsens preexistent cardiac diseases or precipitates de novo cardiac events such as myocardial ischemia, heart failure and symptomatic stenotic or regurgitant valvular diseases. Chronic anemia can also lead to organic heart disease such as ventricular hypertrophy, whereas true high output heart failure rarely results from anemia alone, with the exception of beriberi anemia [22].

Vitamin B deficiency can lead to cardiomyopathy and heart failure in association with megaloblastic anemia in the setting of wet beriberi. It is a very rare disease, mostly seen nowadays in association with tropical sprue and in developing countries [23].

Heart Failure

In patients with heart failure, anemia increases the rate of hospitalization as well as mortality by twofold [1, 24], when compared to those with heart failure alone. It has also been associated with a worse quality of life [25]. A definite causal relationship between anemia and mortality has not been established. A multivariate analysis in a large study of 50 000 chronic heart failure patients did not establish anemia as an independent factor of increased mortality, but rather as an indicator of poor prognosis due to multiple confounding comorbidities [26]. Furthermore, correcting anemia in systolic heart failure with erythropoietin administration did not improve outcome. This supports the idea that anemia is not a direct cause of increased mortality but a surrogate predictor of outcome [27].

Though any type of anemia can be seen in patients with heart failure, iron deficiency anemia is the most common form of anemia encountered in the heart failure population. Even in the absence of anemia, iron deficiency in itself is a poor prognostic factor, leading to reduced exercise capacity and increased mortality in patients with systolic heart failure [28]. Iron deficiency is more common in women, with higher plasma N-terminal pro-brain natriuretic peptide levels and higher serum high-sensitivity C-reactive protein [29]. In addition to the type of anemia, the pattern of anemia evolution was found to have a prognostic role. Persistent anemia after hospital discharge correlates with increased mortality and poorer health status whereas transient anemia does not affect mortality [30].

In patients with assisted ventricular device, the coexistence of anemia also portends a poor prognosis with a marked decrease in one year survival compared to non-hemolyzers (39 % vs 89%, respectively) [31].

Acute Coronary Syndrome

Anemia is a prognostic indicator in patients with ST-elevation myocardial infarction (STEMI). In a retrospective study that included 25000 patients, the adjusted odds ratio of cardiovascular mortality at 30 days after a STEMI was 1.21 for each 1g/dL decrease in hemoglobin below 14g/dL [32]. The highest increase in mortality after STEMI associated with anemia lies within the first 30 days [33]. Long-term mortality up to 24 months may also be increased in patients with anemia on admission or at hospital discharge [34]. The increased mortality and morbidity can be partially explained by less use of antithrombotic, anticoagulants and drug eluted without a delay in the time to balloon duration in anemic patients [3].

In unstable angina and non-ST-elevation myocardial infarction (NSTEMI), the odds that death, myocardial infarction or recurrent ischemia occur, increased when hemoglobin level fell below 11 g/dl [32]. The increased occurrence of adverse events in patients with anemia in the setting of an acute coronary syndrome is most likely explained by the need for oxygen supply to limit myocardial necrosis and penumbral ischemia. Moderate to severe anemia by itself can also cause ischemia by the same mechanism and cause coronary flow insufficiency.

Diagnostic Issues

The usually recommended laboratory tests to diagnose anemia raise several pitfalls in the setting of heart failure. MCV and RDW can be helpful in partially discriminating iron deficiency from inflammatory and hemolytic process. Serum iron and transferrin levels decrease during inflammation. Therefore, their diagnostic role in measuring iron deficiency is limited. Ferritin is the standard biomarker to diagnose iron deficiency in otherwise healthy subjects. Ferritin is also an acute phase reactant; hence, it may be falsely elevated even in the presence of iron deficiency in patients with heart failure [35]. On the other hand, ferritin index can be a useful indicator of the iron supply for erythropoiesis. The ferritin index is the ratio of serum soluble transferrin receptor (sTfR) to the logarithm of serum ferritin level. The index is more specific than ferritin alone since sTfR increases on erythroid precursors regardless of iron stores (which are usually estimated by ferritin) [36]. The sTfR was also found to negatively correlate with the myocardial iron load which is usually low in failing hearts regardless of the level of iron in the serum [37].

The presence of elevated levels of plasma lactate dehydrogenase, bilirubin, free hemoglobin and hemoglobinuria should raise the suspicion of hemolysis especially in the presence of an implanted valve or assisted device and prompt further evaluation with echocardiography.

Treatment

Correcting hematinic deficiencies (iron, vitamin B12, and folic acid) should be considered in patients with heart failure.

Two novel treatments remain controversial: the erythropoeisis stimulating agents and intravenous iron. Transfusion and its precise indications are also a matter of polemic.

Erythropoiesis Stimulating Agents

Erythropoiesis stimulating agents have been assessed in the treatment of anemia in heart failure. Several studies have shown some improved outcome [38-39] but the largest multicenter randomized trial, the Reduction of Events by Darbepoetin Alfa in Heart Failure (RED-HF) [40], has failed to demonstrate any benefit on mortality of darbepoetin-alpha in patients with systolic heart failure and mild to moderate anemia. Lack of benefit of EPO may be partially explained by the preponderant resistance to EPO mechanism. In addition, darbepoetin use was associated with increased ischemic cerebral events and thrombotic events. An analogous phenomenon has been observed while treating anemia in chronic kidney disease with adverse events emerging with the use of EPO. It is however unknown whether these events are directly related to increased hemoglobin level or to EPO-specific side-effects [41]. The continuous EPO receptor activator that was developed to correct anemia in chronic kidney disease [42] has not been studied yet in heart failure patients but it could be useful in addressing the problem of EPO insensitivity in heart failure and might have a different adverse event profile as well.

Intravenous Iron Therapy

Intravenous iron has similarly been associated with a reduction in hospitalizations as well as improvement of functional capacity and ejection fraction [43] but with a higher long-term mortality compared to those who did not receive intravenous iron [44]. In addition, both oral and intravenous iron resulted in the same rise in hematocrit level in IRON-HF study [45]. Thus, intravenous iron supplementation is not currently recommended even in the patients with anemia and heart failure [46].

Transfusion

Transfusion is also a controversial subject in the setting of heart disease. Although anemia negatively affects cardiac perfusion and hemodynamic stability of patients with heart disease, correcting anemia with transfusion does not always improve survival and might sometimes be detrimental. The hemoglobin rise after transfusion increases oxygen delivery but not tissue oxygenation (which may even decrease). RBCs that are stored for transfusion are fragile, stiff and depleted in 2, 3-diphosphoglyceric acid. Transfusion of these cells affects subsequently tissue oxygen extraction and reduces nitric oxide activity leading to less vasodilation during oxygen delivery [47]. In the setting of coronary angioplasty, transfusion is prothrombotic: thus, the concept of treatment-risk paradox well elaborated in the literature [3]. Transfusion induces ADP-P2Y12 receptors leading to platelet activation and aggregation [48]. Stored RBCs have increased levels of procoagulant plasminogen activator inhibitor (PAI)-1 and CD40 ligand platelet release occurs during transfusion [47]. Clinically, there is an increased risk of myocardial ischemia, stroke and in-hospital deaths after RBCs transfusions in patients undergoing a percutaneous coronary intervention as shown by the US CathPCI Registry [49].

The decision to transfuse should be based on symptoms and patient condition rather than on hemoglobin level alone. Patients with cardiovascular diseases are more readily susceptible to develop a decompensate state then those with normal heart, the latter being capable of tolerating a hemoglobin of 5 g/dl before developing myocardial ischemia [3].

In asymptomatic anemic patients with heart failure, a restrictive transfusion strategy at a hemoglobin threshold of 7-8g/dL is recommended more than liberal transfusion at a level <10g/dl [2]. The ACP guidelines adopt the same approach in patients with coronary artery disease. This recommendation is based on low-quality evidence showing no survival improvement with liberal transfusion compared to restrictive transfusion strategy [50]. Moreover, a pilot study of 110 patients with heart failure found a significantly greater 30-day survival with restrictive transfusion strategy at a hemoglobin level <8g/dL than a liberal one at a level <10g/dL [51].

Transfusion at a level <10g/dL is warranted however in severely symptomatic anemia (acute myocardial ischemia, orthostatic hypotension or tachycardia resistant to fluid replacement) whereas exertional symptoms do not justify transfusion.

In conclusion, the exact hemoglobin threshold for transfusion in coronary artery disease patients is still unclear due to the lack of large randomized trials.

The target hemoglobin level is controversial as well. Some studies report a target level of 12-14.9g/dL in patients with heart failure which is remarkably higher than the level of 10-12g/dL retained for CKD [10]. In patients with both chronic kidney disease and heart failure the target is even more uncertain. The CHOIR (Correction of Hemoglobin and Outcomes in Renal Insufficiency) study evaluated the effects of achieving relatively high hemoglobin levels (13.5 g/dl) compared with lower hemoglobin levels (11.3 g/dl) on cardiovascular outcomes in a chronic kidney disease population. This study was prematurely halted because of a surprisingly higher rate of adverse events in the high hemoglobin group [52]. This increase in serious adverse events mainly thrombotic events might be due to high doses of EPO.

In cases of paravalvular leak or thrombus formation on assisted devices, the mainstay of anemia therapy is treatment of the etiology and replacing the prosthetic device.

Conclusion

Anemia occurs in heart failure patients due to the coexistence of inflammation and chronic disease while in those with coronary artery disease it is mostly due to overt or occult bleeding.

The administration of erythropoietin or intravenous iron for asymptomatic patients has not been proven to be beneficial and was associated with increased mortality. In patients with severe and resistant congestive heart failure, the use of subcutaneous erythropoietin and intravenous iron for the treatment of the anemia might have a role in improving outcomes. Evidence has shown in that setting an improvement of cardiac and renal function, functional cardiac class, and reduction in the rate of hospitalizations [53].

The threshold at which transfusion should be considered is controversial, but most societies agree that a hemoglobin <7 g/dl is reasonable in heart failure and chronic ischemic heart disease while hemoglobin <10 g/dl is reasonable in symptomatic anemia leading to myocardial ischemia because of coronary flow insufficiency.

References

[1] Groenveld HF, Januzzi JL, Damman K, van Wijngaarden J, Hillege HL, van Veldhuisen DJ, van der Meer P. Anemia and mortality in heart failure patients a systematic review and meta-analysis. *J. Am. Coll. Cardiol.* 2008;52(10):818-27.

[2] Kansagara D, Dyer E, Englander H, Fu R, Freeman M, Kagen D. Treatment of anemia in patients with heart disease: a systematic review. *Ann. Intern. Med.* 2013;159(11):746-57.

[3] Riley RF, Newby LK, Don CW, Alexander KP, Peterson ED, Peng SA, Gandhi SK, Kutcher MA, Amsterdam EA, Herrington DM. Guidelines-based treatment of anaemic STEMI patients: practice patterns and effects on in-hospital mortality: a retrospective analysis from the NCDR. *Eur. Heart J. Acute Cardiovasc. Care.* 2013 Mar;2(1):35-43.

[4] Weiss G, Goodnough LT. Anemia of chronic disease. *N. Engl. J. Med.* 2005 Mar 10;352(10):1011-23.

[5] Opasich C, Cazzola M, Scelsi L, De Feo S, Bosimini E, Lagioia R, Febo O, Ferrari R, Fucili A, Moratti R, Tramarin R, Tavazzi L. Blunted erythropoietin production and defective iron supply for erythropoiesis as major causes of anaemia in patients with chronic heart failure. *Eur. Heart J.* 2005 Nov;26(21):2232-7.

[6] Belonje AM, Voors AA, van der Meer P, van Gilst WH, Jaarsma T, van Veldhuisen DJ. Endogenous erythropoietin and outcome in heart failure. *Circulation.* 2010 Jan 19;121(2):245-51.

[7] Freudenthaler SM, Schreeb K, Körner T, Gleiter CH. Angiotensin II increases erythropoietin production in healthy human volunteers. *Eur. J. Clin. Invest.* 1999 Oct;29(10):816-23Belonje AM. Circulation 2010.

[8] Smith KJ, Bleyer AJ, Little WC, Sane DC. The cardiovascular effects of erythropoietin. *Cardiovasc Res.* 2003;59: 538 –548.

[9]   Ronco C, House AA, Haapio M. Cardiorenal syndrome: refining the definition of a complex symbiosis gone wrong. *Intensive Care Med.* 2008;34:957–62.
[10] Silverberg DS, Wexler D, Blum M, Keren G, Sheps D, Leibovitch E, Brosh D, Laniado S, Schwartz D, Yachnin T, Shapira I, Gavish D, Baruch R, Koifman B, Kaplan C, Steinbruch S, Iaina A. The use of subcutaneous erythropoietin and intravenous iron for the treatment of the anemia of severe, resistant congestive heart failure improves cardiac and renal function and functional cardiac class, and markedly reduces hospitalizations. *J. Am. Coll. Cardiol.* 2000 Jun;35(7):1737-44.
[11] Hochholzer W, Wiviott SD, Antman EM, Contant CF, Guo J, Giugliano RP, Dalby AJ, Montalescot G, Braunwald E. Predictors of bleeding and time dependence of association of bleeding with mortality: insights from the Trial to Assess Improvement in Therapeutic Outcomes by Optimizing Platelet Inhibition With Prasugrel--Thrombolysis in Myocardial Infarction 38 (TRITON-TIMI 38). *Circulation.* 2011 Jun 14;123(23):2681-9.
[12] Giugliano RP, Giraldez RR, Morrow DA, Antman EM, Gibson CM, Mohanavelu S, Murphy SA, McCabe CH, Braunwald E. Relations between bleeding and outcomes in patients with ST-elevation myocardial infarction in the ExTRACT-TIMI 25 trial. *European Heart Journal* (2010) 31, 2103–2110.
[13] Handelman GJ, Levin NW. Iron and anemia in human biology: a review of mechanisms. *Heart Fail Rev.* 2008 Dec;13(4):393-404.
[14] Ganz T, Nemeth E. Hepcidin and disorders of iron metabolism. *Annu. Rev. Med.* 2011;62:347-60.
[15] Braunwald's Heart Disease: A Textbook of Cardiovascular Medicine, Single Volume, 9th Edition. Robert O. Bonow, MD, Douglas L. Mann, MD, FACC, Douglas P. Zipes, MD and Peter Libby, MD.
[16] Abourjaili G, Torbey E, Alsaghir T, Olkovski Y, Costantino T. Hemolytic anemia following mitral valve repair: A case presentation and literature review. *Exp. Clin. Cardiol.* 2012 Winter;17(4):248-50.
[17] Whitson BA, Eckman P, Kamdar F, Lacey A, Shumway SJ, Liao KK, John R. Hemolysis, pump thrombus, and neurologic events in continuous-flow left ventricular assist device recipients. *Ann. Thorac. Surg.* 2014 Jun; 97(6):2097-103.
[18] Johannsdottir GA, Onundarson PT, Gudmundsdottir BR, Bjornsson ES. Screening for anemia in patients on warfarin facilitates diagnosis of

gastrointestinal malignancies and pre-malignant lesions. *Thromb. Res.* 2012 Sep; 130(3):e20-5.

[19] Crow S, Chen D, Milano C, Thomas W, Joyce L, Piacentino V 3rd, Sharma R, Wu J, Arepally G, Bowles D, Rogers J, Villamizar-Ortiz N. Acquired von Willebrand syndrome in continuous-flow ventricular assist device recipients. *Ann. Thorac. Surg.* 2010 Oct;90(4):1263-9.

[20] Most AS, Ruocco NA Jr, Gewirtz H. Effect of a reduction in blood viscosity on maximal myocardial oxygen delivery distal to a moderate coronary stenosis. *Circulation.* 1986;74:1085–1092.

[21] Levy PS, Quigley RL, Gould SA. Acute dilutional anemia and critical left anterior descending coronary artery stenosis impairs end organ oxygen delivery. *J. Trauma.* 1996;41:416–423.

[22] Porter WB, James GW 3rd. The heart in anemia. *Circulation.* 1953;8(1):111-6.

[23] Cardiovascular beriberi. *Lancet.* 1982 Jun 5;1(8284):1287.

[24] Zuccalà G, Marzetti E, Cesari M, Lo Monaco MR, Antonica L, Cocchi A, Carbonin P, Bernabei R. Correlates of cognitive impairment among patients with heartfailure: results of a multicenter survey. *Am. J. Med.* 2005 May;118(5):496-5023.

[25] Adams KF Jr, Patterson JH, Oren RM, Mehra MR, O'Connor CM, Piña IL, Miller AB, Chiong JR, Dunlap SH, Cotts WG, Felker GM, Schocken DD, Schwartz TA, Ghali JK; STAMINA-HFP Registry Investigators. Prospective assessment of the occurrence of anemia in patients with heart failure: results from the Study of Anemia in a Heart Failure Population (STAMINA-HFP) Registry. *Am. Heart J.* 2009.

[26] Kosiborod M, Curtis JP, Wang Y, Smith GL, Masoudi FA, Foody JM, Havranek EP, Krumholz HM. Anemia and outcomes in patients with heart failure: a study from the National Heart Care Project. *Arch. Intern. Med.* 2005 Oct 24;165(19):2237-44.

[27] Swedberg et al. Treatment of anemia with darbapoetin alfa in systolic heart failure. *N. Engl. J. Med.* 2013;368(13): 1210.

[28] Klip IT, Comin-Colet J, Voors AA, Ponikowski P, Enjuanes C, Banasiak W, Lok DJ, Rosentryt P, Torrens A, Polonski L, van Veldhuisen DJ, van der Meer P, Jankowska EA. Iron deficiency in chronic heart failure: an international pooled analysis. Am Heart J. 2013 Apr;165(4):575-582.e3. Jankowska EA, *Eur. Heart J.* 2010.

[29] Jankowska EA, Rozentryt P, Witkowska A, Nowak J, Hartmann O, Ponikowska B, Borodulin-Nadzieja L, Banasiak W, Polonski L, Filippatos G, McMurray JJ, Anker SD, Ponikowski P. Iron deficiency:

an ominous sign in patients with systolic chronic heart failure. *Eur. Heart J.* 2010 Aug;31(15): 1872-80.
- [30] Salisbury AC, Kosiborod M, Amin AP, Reid KJ, Alexander KP, Spertus JA, Masoudi FA. Recovery from hospital-acquired anemia after acute myocardial infarction and effect on outcomes. *Am. J. Cardiol.* 2011 Oct 1;108(7):949-54.
- [31] Ravichandran AK, Parker J, Novak E, Joseph SM, Schilling JD, Ewald GA, Silvestry S. Hemolysis in left ventricular assist device: a retrospective analysis of outcomes. *J. Heart Lung Transplant.* 2014 Jan;33(1):44-50.
- [32] Sabatine M, Morrow D, Giugliano R, Burton P, Murphy S, McCabe C, C. Michael Gibson CM, Braunwald E. Association of hemoglobin levels with clinical outcomes in acute coronary syndromes. *Braunwald E Circulation.* 2005;111(16):2042.
- [33] Mehran R, Pocock SJ, Stone GW, Clayton TC, Dangas GD, Feit F, Manoukian SV, Nikolsky E, Lansky AJ, Kirtane A, White HD, Colombo A, Ware JH, Moses JW, Ohman EM. Associations of major bleeding and myocardial infarction with the incidence and timing of mortality in patients presenting with non-ST-elevation acute coronary syndromes: a risk model from the ACUITY trial. *Eur. Heart J.* 2009 Jun;30(12):1457-66.
- [34] Aronson D, Suleiman M, Agmon Y, Suleiman A, Blich M, Kapeliovich M, Beyar R, Markiewicz W, Hammerman H. Changes in haemoglobin levels during hospital course and long-term outcome after acute myocardial infarction. *Eur. Heart J.* 2007 Jun;28(11):1289-96.
- [35] Cunietti E, Chiari MM, Monti M, Engaddi I, Berlusconi A, Neri MC, De Luca P. Distortion of iron status indices by acute inflammation in older hospitalized patients. *Arch. Gerontol. Geriatr.* 2004 Jul-Aug;39(1):35-42.
- [36] Means RT Jr, Allen J, Sears DA, Schuster SJ. Serum soluble transferring receptor and the prediction of marrow aspirate iron results in a heterogeneous group of patients. *Clin. Lab. Haematol.* 1999 Jun;21(3):161-7.
- [37] Leszek P, Sochanowicz B, Szperl M, Kolsut P, Brzóska K, Piotrowski W, Rywik TM, Danko B, Polkowska-Motrenko H, Różański JM, Kruszewski M. Myocardial iron homeostasis in advanced chronic heart failure patients. *Int. J. Cardiol.* 2012 Aug 9;159(1):47-52.
- [38] Ponikowski P, Anker SD, Szachniewicz J, Okonko D, Ledwidge M, Zymlinski R, Ryan E, Wasserman SM, Baker N, Rosser D, Rosen SD,

Poole-Wilson PA, Banasiak W, Coats AJ, McDonald K. Effect of darbepoetin alfa on exercise tolerance in anemic patients with symptomatic chronic heart failure: a randomized, double-blind, placebo-controlled trial. *J. Am. Coll. Cardiol.* 2007 Feb 20;49(7):753-62.

[39] Ghali JK, Anand IS, Abraham WT, Fonarow GC, Greenberg B, Krum H, Massie BM, Wasserman SM, Trotman ML, Sun Y, Knusel B, Armstrong P; Study of Anemia in Heart Failure Trial (STAMINA-HeFT) Group. Randomized double-blind trial of darbepoetin alfa in patients with symptomatic heart failure and anemia. *Circulation.* 2008;117(4):526-35.

[40] Swedberg K, Young JB, Anand IS, Cheng S, Desai AS, Diaz R, Maggioni AP, McMurray JJ, O'Connor C, Pfeffer MA, Solomon SD, Sun Y, Tendera M, van Veldhuisen DJ; RED-HF Committees; RED-HF Investigators. Treatment of anemia with darbepoetin alfa in systolic heart failure. *N. Engl. J. Med.* 2013;368(13):1210-9.

[41] Kazory A, Ross E. Anemia: the point of convergence or divergence for kidney disease and heart failure? *J. Am. Coll. Cardiol.* 2009;53:639-47.

[42] Macdougall IC, Walker R, Provenzano R, de Alvaro F, Locay HR, Nader PC, Locatelli F, Dougherty FC, Beyer U; ARCTOS Study Investigators. C.E.R.A. corrects anemia in patients with chronic kidney disease not on dialysis: results of a randomized clinical trial. *Clin. J. Am. Soc. Nephrol.* 2008 Mar;3(2):337-47.

[43] Kapoor M, Schleinitz MD, Gemignani A, Wu WC. Outcomes of patients with chronic heart failure and iron deficiency treated with intravenous iron: a meta-analysis. *Cardiovasc. Hematol. Disord. Drug Targets.* 2013 Mar 1;13(1):35-44.

[44] Besarab A, Bolton WK, Browne JK, Egrie JC, Nissenson AR, Okamoto DM, Schwab SJ, Goodkin DA. The effects of normal as compared with low hematocrit values in patients with cardiac disease who are receiving hemodialysis and epoetin. *N. Engl. J. Med.* 1998 Aug 27;339(9):584-90.

[45] Beck-da-Silva L, Piardi D, Soder S, Rohde LE, Pereira-Barretto AC, de Albuquerque D, Bocchi E, Vilas-Boas F, Moura LZ, Montera MW, Rassi S, Clausell N.IRON-HF study: a randomized trial to assess the effects of iron in heart failure patients with anemia. *Int. J. Cardiol.* 2013 Oct 9;168(4):3439-42.

[46] Arora Np, Ghali JK. Anemia and iron deficiency in heart failure. *Heart Failure Clin.* 2014 Apr;10 (2):281-94.

[47] Hajjar LA, Vincent JL, Galas FR, Nakamura RE, Silva CM, Santos MH, Fukushima J, Kalil Filho R, Sierra DB, Lopes NH, Mauad T, Roquim

AC, Sundin MR, Leão WC, Almeida JP, Pomerantzeff PM, Dallan LO, Jatene FB, Stolf NA, Auler JO Jr. Transfusion requirements after cardiac surgery: the TRACS randomized controlled trial. *JAMA.* 2010 Oct 13;304(14):1559-67.

[48] Silvain J, Abtan J, Kerneis M, Martin R, Finzi J, Vignalou JB, Barthélémy O, O'Connor SA, Luyt CE, Brechot N, Mercadier A, Brugier D, Galier S, Collet JP, Chastre J, Montalescot G. Impact of red blood cell transfusion on platelet aggregation and inflammatory response in anemic coronary and noncoronary patients: the TRANSFUSION-2 study (impact of transfusion of red blood cell on platelet activation and aggregation studied with flow cytometry use and light transmission aggregometry). *J. Am. Coll. Cardiol.* 2014 Apr 8;63(13): 1289-96.

[49] Sherwood MW, Wang Y, Curtis JP, Peterson ED, Rao SV. Patterns and outcomes of red blood cell transfusion in patients undergoing percutaneous coronary intervention. *JAMA.* 2014 Feb 26;311(8):836-43.

[50] Qaseem A, Humphrey LL, Fitterman N, Starkey M, Shekelle P; Clinical Guidelines Committee of the American College of Physicians. Treatment of anemia in patients with heart disease: a clinical practice guideline from the American College of Physicians. *Ann. Intern. Med.* 2013 Dec 3;159(11):770-9.

[51] Carson JL, Brooks MM, Abbott JD, Chaitman B, Kelsey SF, Triulzi DJ, Srinivas V, Menegus MA, Marroquin OC, Rao SV, Noveck H, Passano E, Hardison RM, Smitherman T, Vagaonescu T, Wimmer NJ, Williams DO. Liberal versus restrictive transfusion thresholds for patients with symptomatic coronary artery disease. *Am. Heart J.* 2013 Jun;165(6):964-971.

[52] Singh AK, Szczech L, Tang KL, Barnhart H, Sapp S, Wolfson M, Reddan D; CHOIR Investigators. Correction of anemia with epoetin alfa in chronic kidney disease. *N. Engl. J. Med.* 2006 Nov 16;355(20):2085-98.

[53] Reinecke H, Trey T, Wellmann J, Heidrich J, Fobker M, Wichter T, Walter M, Breithardt G, Schaefer RM. Haemoglobin-related mortality in patients undergoing percutaneous coronary interventions. *Eur. Heart J.* 2003 Dec; 24(23):2142-50.

In: Anemia
Editor: Alice Hallman

ISBN: 978-1-63321-775-1
© 2014 Nova Science Publishers, Inc.

Chapter 2

Influence of Iron Deficiency Anaemia and Recovery on Oxidative/Antioxidant Status

Javier Díaz-Castro[1,2,*], Mario Pulido-Moran[1,3], Silvia Hijano[1,2], Naroa Kajarabille[1,2] and Julio J. Ochoa[1,2]
[1]Institute of Nutrition and Food Technology "José Mataix Verdú",
Biomedical Research Center, University of Granada, Granada, Spain
[2]Departament of Physiology, Faculty of Pharmacy, Campus de Cartuja,
University of Granada, Granada, Spain
[3]Departament of Biochemistry and Molecular Biology II,
Faculty of Pharmacy, Campus de Cartuja,
University of Granada, Granada, Spain

Abstract

Oxidative stress results from an imbalance between the formation and neutralization of ROS and it is imposed on cells as a result of one or more of the following factors: an increase in oxidant generation, a decrease in antioxidant protection, or a failure to repair oxidative damage.

---

[*] Corresponding author: Department of Physiology and Institute of Nutrition and Food Technology, University of Granada, Biomedical Research Centre, Health Sciences Technological Park, Avenida del Conocimiento s/n, Armilla, 18071 Granada, Spain, Tel.: +34 958241000 ext. 20303. E-mail address: javierdc@ugr.es

There is controversy about the susceptibility of cells to lipid peroxidation in Fe deficiency anaemia: some investigators have claimed there is no difference in lipid peroxidation among patients with Fe deficiency anaemia compared with controls, but others have reported that among patients with IDA oxidants are increased and antioxidants decreased, so the oxidative/antioxidative balance is shifted toward the oxidative side. This apparent discrepancy may be due to different concentrations of ROS and antioxidant enzymes in the tissues studied, the subjects of the study, the severity of the Fe-deficiency and the methods used for the assessment of the oxidative stress. However, in humans, were the degree of Fe-deficiency is not very high, it is accepted that Fe-deficiency increases oxidative stress, fact that can also be attributed to the repletion process with several sources of Fe. Several authors have reported increased lipid peroxidation products in patients with Fe deficiency anaemia, which may be attributed to over production of ROS and a deficiency of antioxidant defense. Decreased SOD activity in Fe deficiency anaemia may be linked to increased oxidative stress, because it is well known that ROS, inhibit SOD activity. Other authors also found that CAT activity was significantly decreased in Fe-deficiency groups as compared with controls. CAT is an iron-dependent enzyme and is not unexpected to be decreased in iron deficiency.

1. Introduction

1.1. Oxidative Stress

Oxidative stress results from an imbalance between the formation and neutralization of oxygen-derived pro-oxidants, which can cause damage to biological targets such as lipids, DNA, and proteins, and on the defending systems of the cell, which are composed of enzymes and reducing equivalents, or antioxidants. In general these pro-oxidants are referred to as reactive oxygen species (ROS) that can be classified into 2 groups of compounds, radicals and nonradicals. The radical group, often incorrectly called free-radical (the term is not accurate, because a radical is always free.), contains compounds such as nitric oxide radical (NO·), superoxide ion radical (O_2^-), hydroxyl radical (OH·), peroxyl (ROO·) and alkoxyl radicals (RO·), and one form of singlet oxygen ($^1O_2$). These species are radicals, because they contain at least 1 unpaired electron in the shells around the atomic nucleus and are capable of independent existence (Halliwell and Gutteridge, 1999; Kohen and Niska, 2002; Rice-Evans and Burdon, 2004).

Most of the transition metals contain unpaired electrons and can, therefore, with the exception of zinc, be considered radicals by definition (Halliwell and Gutteridge, 1999). They can participate in the chemistry of radicals and convert relatively stable oxidants into powerful radicals. Among the various transition metals, copper and especially iron aremost abundant, present in relatively high concentrations, and are major players in the Fenton reaction (Fenton, 1984) and the metal-mediated Haber-Weiss reaction (Haber and Weiss, 1934). The metal ions participating in this reaction are those bound to the surface of proteins, DNA, and other macromolecules or chelates. These particular ions can still undergo the reduction-oxidation process, interact with oxygen derivatives, and are often called "loosely bound metals" or "removable metals" (Sutton and Winterbourn, 1989). Metals that are hidden in proteins, as in catalytic sites and cytochromes, or storage complexes; are not exposed to oxygen radicals; or are kept under 1 oxidation state cannot participate in this chemistry.

1.1. Iron Deficiency Anaemia

Iron deficiency is extremely common in humans, and is the most widespread nutritional deficiency in the world. To more fully understand iron deficiency anemia, consideration must be directed toward concepts of iron supply and demand for the production of erythrocytes. Erythropoiesis-related demands for iron are created by three variables: tissue oxygenation, erythrocyte turnover, and erythrocyte loss from hemorrhage. Tissue oxygenation requirements and erythrocyte production generally remain stable during adulthood in the absence of hemorrhage, disease, or altered physical activity.

The most affected groups are women in fertile age, especially pregnant women and children, during the stage of growth. Anaemia takes place when the levels of Fe decrease or the requirements overcome the contribution of the intake that is provided in the diet, so the Fe storages of the organism are depleted. There is no doubt that the Fe deficiency is the major cause of the great majority of anaemias. The Fe-deficiency anaemia is characterized by low levels of serum Fe and haemoglobin (Hb), reduction of the haematocrit and increased levels of platelets (Campos et al., 1998), low percentage of transferrin saturation, decrease of serum ferritin and a drastic increase in total Fe binding capacity (TIBC) (Díaz-Castro et al., 2013).

In addition, the chemical properties of Fe render it a potential hazard within the organism in that ferrous ion Fe (II), in small non-protein shielded chelates, can catalyze the production of reactive oxygen species (ROS), which in turn can lead to peroxidation and radical chain reactions with molecular damage (Aust and Eveleigh, 1999; Haliwell et al., 2011).

On the other hand, regulation of ROS levels and oxidative stress is extremely important in erythropoiesis. Starting at the basophilic erythroblast stage, erythroid precursors synthesize large amounts of Hb, which require haem as a prosthetic group.

Thus, Fe uptake for haem biosynthesis also increases, potentially generating ROS through the Fenton reaction (Ghaffari, 2008).

Oxidative stress results from an imbalance between the formation and neutralization of ROS and it is imposed on cells as a result of one or more of the following factors: an increase in oxidant generation, a decrease in antioxidant protection, or a failure to repair oxidative damage (Aust and Eveleigh, 1999; Haliwell et al., 2011). Disturbance of the pro-oxidant/antioxidant balance is also considered to be a causative factor underlying oxidative damage to cellular molecules, such as DNA, causing strand breaks.

There is controversy about the susceptibility of cells to lipid peroxidation in Fe deficiency anaemia: some investigators have claimed there is no difference in lipid peroxidation among patients with Fe deficiency anaemia compared with controls (Acharya et al., 1991; Isler et al., 2002), but others have reported that among patients with IDA oxidants are increased and antioxidants decreased, so the oxidative/antioxidative balance is shifted toward the oxidative side (Vives corrons et al., 1995; Kumerova et al., 1998; Aslan et al., 2006).

In a study by Díaz-Castro et al. (2008), the authors reported that Fe deficiency anaemia does not affect DNA stability or lipid peroxidation in rats and suggest that there is enough compensatory capacity to keep antioxidant defenses high.

This apparent discrepancy may be due to different concentrations of ROS and antioxidant enzymes in the tissues studied, the subjects of the study, the severity of the Fe-deficiency and the methods used for the assessment of the oxidative stress. However, in humans, were the degree of Fe-deficiency is not very high, it is accepted that Fe-deficiency increases lipid peroxidation, fact that can also be attributed to the repletion process with several sources of Fe.

2. Influence of Iron Deficiency Anaemia on Oxidative/Antioxidant Status, DNA Stability and Lipid Peroxidation

The DNA repair system is a cellular defence mechanism responding to DNA damage caused in large part by oxidative stress. The DNA damaging agents are either external, such as pollution and exposure to sunshine or other types of irradiation, or internal such as a consequence of replication or metabolic pathways that produce reactive oxygen species (ROS). It has been observed that red blood cells (RBC) may affect the DNA damage and repair system. The active substance may be either the whole hemoglobin molecule or the ferrum component or other metabolites, such as adenosine phosphate, which exist in RBC. The published effects of whole RBC or RBC hemolysate are contradictive: some investigators did not find any association between DNA damage and hemoglobin (Aksu et al., 2010), others found that hemoglobin caused DNA damage similar to the effect of H_2O_2 (Thorlaksdottir et al., 2007; Park et al., 2011), and another group found a negative correlation between hemoglobin level and DNA damage (Aslan et al., 2006). Porto et al. showed that RBC protected cultured lymphocytes against chromosome breakage induced by the alkylating agent diepoxybutane. This effect was attributed to the RBC hemolysate and hemoglobin, while RBC membrane had no effect (Porto et al., 2003). In a study by Gafter-Gvili et al. (2013), they found that RBC, RBC hemolysate and hemoglobin reduced DNA repair ability in PBMC following H_2O_2-induced DNA breaks. The effect of the RBC hemolysate was dose-dependent. Furthermore, we observed a significant negative correlation between hemoglobin and DNA repair at the concentration of 2% v/v hemolysate. No correlation was seen with lower concentrations of hemolysate. The reduction in DNA repair by RBC, RBC hemolysate and hemoglobin could be due either to their direct effect on the DNA repair reaction or to a defensive effect against H_2O_2-induced DNA damage with the appropriate DNA repair response. Indeed, we have previously seen that the rise in DNA damage due to oxidative stress during dialysis was accompanied by a rise in DNA repair (Tanaka et al., 2006).

The results of Gafter-Gvili et al. (2013), are in accordance with the studies which found a negative correlation between hemoglobin level and DNA damage (Aslan et al., 2006), and with the studies that showed protection by normal RBC (Porto et al., 2003) or fetal RBC (Proto et al., 2006) of lymphocytes against chromosomal breakage induced in lymphocytes by the alkylating agent diepoxybutane. Similar to these findings, Porto et al. suggested that this effect is obtained by hemolysed RBC and more specifically by the hemoglobin (Porto et al., 2003). They further suggested an additional protective effect of fetal RBC due to increased antioxidative activity by the increased glutathione transferase, catalase and superoxide dismutase activity in fetal RBC (Porto et al., 2006).

Diaz-Castro et al. (2008) reported that the susceptibility of the hepatic cytosolic fraction in animals Fe-deficient models did not significantly differ from control non anaemic animals and nor differences were found in liver GSH-Px antioxidant enzyme activity. DNA oxidative damage was not affected in Fe-defient rats. It has been reported that GSH-Px activity in anemia is similar to that of normal cells (Acharya et al., 1991; Isler et al., 2002). The GSH-Px activity in the study of Díaz-Castro et al., 2008 was in accordance with the results reported by these investigators and in contrast to those of many others (Vives corrons et al., 1995; Kumerova et al., 1998; Aslan et al., 2006). No correlations were found between Fe concentration and GSH-Px. It is well known that Fe is not the only cause of changes in GSH-Px activity in patients with Fe-deficiency anaemia; other minerals, such as selenium, copper, zinc, and manganese, which mediate the activities of these enzymes, may also play an important role in the alteration of enzyme radicals via Fenton and Haber-Weiss chemistries, which explains and supports the lack of differences between control and anaemic rats regarding lipid peroxidation (Díaz-Castro et al., 2008).

Oxidative status in Fe-deficency anaemia has been widely investigated (although the results obtained have been ambiguous), but there is little information concerning DNA damage. Diaz-Castro et al. (2008) reported that lymphocyte DNA damage was not increased by Fe deficiency. Iron deficiency induces changes in the cellular Fe homeostasis system. Dietary Fe deficiency causes an increase in liver iron responsive element binding protein-1 activity, which increases transferrin receptor synthesis and decreases mitochondrial–aconitase activity. The decrease in mitochondrial–aconitase activity may prevent further mitochondrial release of oxidants by diminishing the supply of reducing equivalents to the electron-transport chain. The reduced electron flow may be one way by which the cell protects itself from oxidant stress in Fe deficiency (Chen et al., 1997). Furthermore, Fe excess promotes the generation of oxygen radicals (especially hydroxyl radicals via Fenton and Haber- Weiss reactions), which may cause oxidative damage such as the degradation of DNA, causing strand breaks (Aust and Eveleigh, 1999), so Fe deficiency could exert a protective effect, preventing, at least in part, the generation of free radicals, and the subsequent DNA damage. Cragg et al. (Craig et al., 1998) examined the effects of hydrogen peroxide on HepG2 cells and showed that the Fe loading greatly exacerbates the DNA damage induced by hydrogen peroxide and that a Fe chelator (desferrithiocin) exerts a protective effect on the cells. These facts can explain the findings of Diaz-Castro et al. (2008) regarding the stability of lymphocyte DNA.

In other study, however, it has been reported that severely anemic, iron-deficient rats, as well as rats supplemented daily with high iron, were shown previously to have increased lipid peroxidation, as indicated by elevated levels of malondialdehyde in liver and kidney and ethane in breath (Knutson et al., 2000). Another study shows that iron deficiency increased oxidant levels in polymorphonuclear leukocytes and liver mtDNA damage. Iron deficiency also decreased liver mitochondrial RCR, a measure of respiratory efficiency (Walter et al., 2000). Walter et al. (2000) proposed four possible mechanisms by which iron deficiency can cause damage to mitochondria and its DNA:

a) The uncoupling of mitochondria can increase mitochondrial superoxide release (45), probably due to decreased heme availability. Decreased cytochrome concentration of the electron-transport chain could also possibly contribute to increased superoxide levels. The increased superoxide released from these uncoupled mitochondria could account for the observed elevation of liver peroxidation and, mtDNA damage.

b) Gastrointestinal up-regulation of iron absorption during iron deficiency increases copper absorption and hepatic copper accumulation in rats. The increased copper absorption may be mediated by divalent metal transporter 1 (DMT1), which is dramatically up-regulated in iron-deficient duodenum. Copper can participate in Fenton chemistry with H_2O_2 generating reactive hydroxyl radicals that can damage lipids and DNA. Moreover, excess copper can cause severe mitochondrial dysfunction and mtDNA damage, as has been reported in the livers of patients with copper overload caused by Wilson's disease.

c) Iron deficiency causes loss of activity of some important iron-containing repair enzymes. For example, the activity of ribonucleotide reductase is decreased in iron-deficient cell cultures; this could lead to decreased availability of deoxyribonucleotides for DNA repair. Treatment of cell cultures with desferrioxamine lowered iron levels as well as dNTPs and DNA synthesis.

d) Iron deficiency also induces changes in the cellular iron homeostasis system. First, dietary iron deficiency causes an increase in liver IRP1 activity, which increases transferrin receptor synthesis. However, ever, after 3 weeks of iron deficiency, IRP1 activity is increased and there is a marked decrease in ferritin synthesis, thus decreasing its potential as an antioxidant protein. Up-regulatio of transferrin receptor (TFR) first maintains or increases cytosolic iron availability in the face of the initial iron deficiency. At the same time, decreasing iron supply may induce an increase in intracellular iron trafficking from iron stores in ferritin and hemosiderin. Therefore, there is an increase in the potential for iron availability to catalyze some of the oxidant-induced damage.

Díaz-Castro et al. (2011) reported a higher Se retention (essential cofactor in GPx) in anemic rats, which resulted from the lower fecal and especially lower urinary excretion. However, a decrease in Se content was found in sternum of anemic rats, which could be explained, at least in part, by the lower count of RBCs. It has been reported that selenite is incorporated into RBC's via an anion-exchange protein expressed in the plasma membrane of these cells (Suzuki et al., 1998). Due to the supply of the Fe-restrictive diet, rats were deeply anemic at the end of the experimental period, reason why it was observed a decrease of Se content in sternum of anemic rats, caused by the Fe depletion and the impaired hematopoiesis, which leads to a decrease on the RBCs count.

Se metabolism has been partly described and comprehensive reviews have shown the biological transformation of Se from inorganic Se compounds and selenoamino acids in foods, into excreted selenocompounds via key metabolic intermediates (Suzuki et al., 2005). The biotransformation of selenite is explained as follows: selenite passively diffuses into the intestine and predominantly exists in bloodstream in spite of the partial transformation into glutathione and/or cysteine conjugated forms in the intestine (Park et al., 2004). Then, selenite is taken up by red blood cells (RBCs) and reduced by abundant glutathione into selenide (Suzuki et al., 1998). During the induced Fe deficiency anemia, the impaired hematopoiesis provokes a diminishing on the RBCs count, leading to an increase of selenite (not reduced) in plasma, which could be bound to albumin and transported to organs and stored in liver, spleen, muscles and testes. Se uptake by the liver was more efficiently in anemic rats, and was supposed to be utilized for the synthesis of selenoproteins. In order to find out how the selenoproteins were affected during the anemia, the liver GPx activity was similar in control and anaemic animals. Because of the hierarchy in Se distribution, the liver is among the first Se pools and cellular GPx the first selenoprotein to be affected in Se depletion (Behne et al., 2001). An unchanged enzymatic activity of the liver GPx is therefore an indication of a normal body status of the other selenoproteins (Díaz-Castro et al., 2011).

3. Influence of Iron Replenishment on Oxidative Stress during Anaemia Recovery

Diaz-Castro et al. (2013) revealed that after 30 days of supplying diets with different Fe sources and amounts, the background DNA damage in the lymphocytes of the peripheral blood was much lower in anaemic rats given the haem Fe (12 mg Fe/kg diet) in comparison with $FeSO_4$ (45 mg Fe/kg diet). Lipid peroxidation in rats was similar in liver, brain and erythrocyte and , except in the duodenal mucosa in which lipid peroxidation was lower in dudodenal mucosa with the diets containing haem Fe (12 mg Fe/kg diet) and $FeSO_4$+haem Fe (31 mg Fe/kg diet). The oxidative protein damage was also lower in anaemic rats fed haem Fe (12 mg Fe/kg diet) in comparison with $FeSO_4$ (45 mg Fe/kg diet).

The lower lipid peroxidation found in the duodenal mucosa of anaemic animals fed with haem Fe (12 mg Fe/kg diet) can be explained partly by the lower amount of free Fe in these diets compared with the diet containing $FeSO_4$ (45 mg Fe/kg diet). But there are other facts that can explain the protective effect in terms of lipid damage with haem Fe. The feedback mechanisms that control Fe absorption and trafficking include several Fe regulatory proteins such as divalent metal transporter 1, transferrin and ferritin between many others. This regulatory function is mediated by Fe responsive elements, which would better recovered with the supply of haem Fe, because haem internalization involves either direct transport of haem or receptor-mediated endocytosis (West and Oates, 2008) in a very efficient process, limiting the Fe available to catalyze ROS generation. Meanwhile, non-haem Fe provided by $FeSO_4$ would result in an excessive Fe trafficking in the intestinal lumen which, in turn, readily attacks and damages cellular lipids, because of its low solubility and high toxicity (Hider et al., 2010).

Oxidative protein damage is higher in the anaemic rats fed FeSO$_4$, revealing that liver proteins are particularly vulnerable to oxidative stress due to the non-haem Fe absorption. This produces a high expression of hepcidin, blocking the liberation of Fe in the hepatocytes (Ben-Assa et al., 2009) in a physiological compensatory mechanism directed to replenish the storage exhausted during the experimentally induced Fe-deficiency. These Fe accumulation storages in the liver would induce the oxidative damage to the proteins.

The protein oxidative damage in erythrocytes was also lower with haem Fe. Under physiological conditions, hydrogen peroxide produced by autooxidation of Fe is a predominant ROS in red blood cells. If this H$_2$O$_2$ is not scavenged immediately by antioxidant defence enzymes, it oxidizes Hb to the higher oxidation state of ferryl-Hb and oxoferryl-Hb, which can cause lipid peroxidation and subsequent oxidative stress including protein and DNA damage (Gil et al., 2006).

Additionally, the haem Fe diet showed lower erythrocyte protein damage probably due to the low amount of free Fe supplied, minimizing Fe plasma trafficking, thus, a low rate of ROS generation that diminishes the rate of autooxidation of free Fe, and avoiding the evoked oxidative stress with classical supplements based on Fe overload.

The brain is unique among all the organs of the body, hidden behind the relatively poorly permeable vascular barrier, which limits its access to plasma nutrients, such as Fe (Crichton et al., 2011). The endothelial cells make up the blood–brain barrier and express transferrin receptor 1 on the luminal side of the capillaries.

These receptors do not increase their expression in Fe deficiency or overload (Moos et al., 2007); therefore, the nervous tissue is relatively independent of the Fe variations in the organism as we previously reported (Díaz-Castro et al., 2012), which is the reason why lipid peroxidation or protein damage did not differ.

Kumar et al. (2010) reported increased lipid peroxidation products in pregnant women with Fe deficiency anaemia, which may be attributed to over production of ROS or a deficiency of antioxidant defense. Antioxidant enzymes are the major defense system of cells in normal aerobic reactions. Although, erythrocytes possess highly efficient antioxidant enzymes, such as CuZn–SOD and GPx compared to other cell types (Kumerova et al., 1998), though as the results showed that women with Fe deficiency anaemia have lower CuZn–SOD activity than healthy control. The results of Diaz-Castro et al. (2008) are in accordance with earlier such reports (Kurtoglu et al., 2003).

Decreased SOD activity in Fe deficiency anaemia may be linked to increased oxidative stress, because it is well known that ROS, especially hydrogen peroxide (H_2O_2), inhibit SOD activity (Isler et al., 2002). CAT and SOD are metaloproteins and accomplish their antioxidant function by enzymatically detoxifying the peroxides. CAT has been suggested to provide important pathway for H2O2 decomposition into H_2O and O_2. Kumar et al. (2010) also found that CAT activity was significantly decreased in IDA groups as compared with controls.

This finding was in agreement with those of Acharya et al. (1991) who also reported decreased CAT activity in patients with Fe deficiency anaemia. CAT is an iron-dependent enzyme and is not unexpected to be decreased in iron deficiency. Similarly, GPx activity in IDA groups was decreased when compared with controls.

This finding is in accordance with the finding of Yetgin et al. (1992), who reported decreased GPx activity in children with iron deficiency. Decreased activity in IDA may be due to perturbed pentose phosphate pathway, as IDA may have restricted the availability of NADPH, a co-factor for GPx functioning (Kumerova et al., 1998). GSH plays a pivotal role in protection of cells against oxidative stress.

It can act as a non-enzymatic antioxidant by direct interactions of SH group with ROS or it can be involved in the enzymatic detoxification reactions for ROS as a coenzyme (Ding et al., 2000).

In the study of Kumar et al. (2010) they also observed significantly depletion of GSH in all anemic groups when compared with control. Significant perturbations were also observed in the oxidized form of GSH, i.e., GSSG. At the same time it must be considered that ferrous iron-used for oral iron therapy is a potent pro-oxidant, increasing the evoked oxidative stress (Díaz-Castro et al., 2013).

Conclusion

In conclusion, there is controversy about the susceptibility of cells to lipid peroxidation in Fe deficiency anaemia: some investigators have claimed there is no difference in lipid peroxidation among patients with Fe deficiency anaemia compared with controls, but others have reported that among patients with Fe-deficiency anaemia oxidants are increased and antioxidants decreased, so the oxidative/antioxidative balance is shifted toward the oxidative side. However, in humans, were the degree of Fe-deficiency is not very high, it is accepted that Fe-deficiency increases oxidative stress, fact that can also be attributed to the repletion process with several sources of Fe. Available data indicate that oxidative stress is higher and total antioxidant and antioxidant enzymes activities are higher after rather than before treatment in patients with Fe-deficiency anaemia.

References

Acharya J, Punchard NA, Taylor IA, Tompson RPH, Peason TC (1991) Red cell peroxidation and antioxidant enzymes in iron deficiency. *Eur. J. Haematol* 47:287–291.

Aksu BY, Hasbal C, Himmetoglu S, Dincer Y, Koc EE, Hatipoglu S, Akcay T (2010) Leukocyte DNA damage in children with iron deficiency anemia: effect of iron supplementation. *Eur. J. Pediatr* 169:951–956.

Tiwari AK, Mahdi AA, Zahra F, Chandyan S, Srivastava VK, Negi MP (2010) Evaluation of Oxidative Stress and Antioxidant Status in Pregnant Anemic Women. *Indian J. Clin. Biochem.* 25(4): 411–418.

Aslan M, Horoz M, Kocyigit A, Ozgonu S, Celik H et al. (2006) Lymphocyte DNA damage and oxidative stress in patients with iron deficiency anemia. *Mutat. Res.* 601: 144–149.

Aust AE, Eveleigh JF (1999) Mechanisms of DNA oxidation. *Proc. Soc. Exp. Biol. Med.* 222:246–252.

Behne D, Kyriakopoulos A (2001) Mammalian selenium-containing proteins. *Annu. Rev. Nutr.* 21:453–473.

Ben-Assa E, Youngster I, Kozer E, Abu-Kishk I, Bar-Haim A, Bar- Oz B, Berkovitch M (2009) Changes in serum hepcidin levels in acute iron intoxication in a rat model. *Toxicol. Lett.* 189:242–247.

Campos MS, Barrionuevo M, Alférez MJM, Gómez-Ayala AE, Rodríguez-Matas MC, López-Aliaga I, Lisbona F (1998) Interactions among iron, calcium, phosphorus and magnesium in nutritionally iron deficient rats. *Exp. Physiol.* 83:771–781.

Chen OS, Schalinske KL, Eisenstein RS (1997) Dietary iron intake modulates the activity of iron regulatory proteins and the abundance of ferritin and mitochondrial aconitase in rat liver. *J. Nutr.* 127:238–48.

Cragg L, Hebel RP, Miller W, Solovey A, Selbey S, Enright H (1998) The iron chelator L1 potentiates oxidative DNA damage in iron-loaded liver cells. *Blood* 92:632–638.

Crichton RR, Dexter DT, Ward RJ (2011) Brain iron metabolism and its perturbation in neurological diseases. *J Neural Transm* 118:301–314.

Díaz-Castro J, Alférez MJ, López-Aliaga I, Nestares T, Granados S, Barrionuevo M, Campos MS (2008) Influence of nutritional iron deficiency anemia on DNA stability and lipid peroxidation in rats. *Nutrition* 24(11-12):1167–11673.

Díaz-Castro J, García Y, López-Aliaga I, Alférez MJ, Hijano S, Ramos A, Campos MS (2013) Influence of several sources and amounts of iron on DNA, lipid and protein oxidative damage during anaemia recovery. *Biol. Trace Elem. Res.* 155(3):403–410.

Díaz-Castro J, Pérez-Sánchez LJ, Ramírez López-Frías M, López- Aliaga I, Nestares T, Alférez MJ, Ojeda ML, Campos MS (2012) Influence of cow or goat milk consumption on antioxidant defence and lipid peroxidation during chronic iron repletion. *Br. J. Nutr.* 108:1–8

Ding Y, Gonick HC, Vaziri ND (2000) Lead promotes hydroxyl radical generation and lipid peroxidation in cultured aortic endothelial cells. *Am. J. Hypertens* 13:552–555.

Fenton HJH (1894). The oxidation of tartaric acid in the presence of iron. *J. Chem. Soc. Proc.* 10:157–158.

Gafter-Gvili A1, Zingerman B, Rozen-Zvi B, Ori Y, Green H, Lubin I, Malachi T, Gafter U, Herman-Edelstein M (2013) Oxidative stress-induced DNA damage and repair in human peripheral blood mononuclear cells: protective role of hemoglobin. *PLoS One* 8(7):e68341.

Ghaffari S (2008) Oxidative stress in the regulation of normal and neoplastic hematopoiesis. *Antioxid Redox Signal* 10:1923–1940.

Gil L, Siems W, Mazurek B, Gross J, Schroeder P, Voss P, Grune T (2006) Age-associated analysis of oxidative stress parameters in human plasma and erythrocytes. *Free Rad. Res.* 40:495–505.

Haber F, Weiss J (1934). The catalytic decomposition of hydrogen peroxide by iron salts. *Proc. R Soc.* London 147:332–351.

Halliwell B, Gutteridge JM (1999) *Free Radicals in Biology and Medicine, third edition.* Oxford University Press, Midsomer Norton, Avon, England.

Halliwell B. (2001) Role of free radicals in neurodegenerative diseases: therapeutic implications for antioxidant treatment. *Drugs Aging* 18:685–716.

Hider RC, Kong XL (2010) Chemistry and biology of siderophores. *Nat. Prod. Rep* 27:637–657.

Isler M, Delibas N, Guclu M, Gultekin F, Sutcu R, Bahceci M, Kosar A (2002) Superoxide dismutase and glutathione peroxidase in erythrocytes of patients with iron deficiency anemia: effects of different treatment modalities. *Croat Med. J.* 43(1):16–19.

Knutson MD, Walter PB, Ames BN, Viteri FE (2000) Both iron deficiency and daily iron supplements increase lipid peroxidation in rats. *J. Nutr.* 130:621–628.

Kohen R, Nyska A (2002) Oxidation of biological systems: oxidative stress phenomena, antioxidants, redox reactions, and methods for their quantification. *Toxicol. Pathol.* 30(6):620–650.

Kumerova A, Lece A, Skesters A, Silova A, Petuhovs V (1998) Anaemia and antioxidant defence of the red blood cells. *Mater. Med. Pol.* 30:2–15.

Kurtoglu E, Ugur A, Baltaci AK, Undar L (2003) Effect of supplementation on oxidative stress and antioxidant status in iron deficiency anemia. *Biol. Trace Elem. Res.* 96:117–123.

Moos T, Rosengren NT, Skjørringe T, Morgan EH (2007) Iron trafficking inside the brain. *J. Neurochem* 103:1730–1740.

Park JH, Park E (2011) Influence of iron-overload on DNA damage and its repair in human leucocytes in vitro. *Mutat. Res.* 718:56–61.

Park YC, Kim JB, Heo Y, Park DC, Lee IS, Chung HW, Han JH, Chung WG, Vendeland SC, Whanger PD (2004) Metabolism of subtoxic level of selenite by double-perfused small intestine in rats. *Biol. Trace Elem. Res.* 98:143–157.

Parkkila S, Niemela O, Savolainen ER, Koistinen P (2001) HFE mutations do not account for transfusional iron overload in patients with acute myeloid leukemia. *Transfusion* 41:828–831.

Walter PB, Knutson MD, Paler-Martinez A, Lee S, Xu Y, Viteri FE, Ames BN (2002) Iron deficiency and iron excess damage mitochondria and mitochondrial DNA in rats. *Proc. Natl. Acad. Sci. U S A* 99(4):2264–2269.

Porto B, Chiecchio L, Gaspar J, Faber A, Pinho L, Rueff J, Malheiro I (2003) Role of haemoglobin in the protection of cultured lymphocytes against diepoxybutane (DEB), assessed by in vitro induced chromosome breakage. *Mutat. Res.* 536: 61–67.

Porto B, Oliveira RJD, Sousa C, Gaspar J, Rueff J, Carvalho F, Malheiro I (2006) The role of foetal red blood cells in protecting cultured lymphocytes against diepoxybutaneinduced chromosome breaks. *Mutat. Res.* 603:41–47.

Rice-Evans CA, Burdon RH (1994) New Comprehensive Biochemistry: Free Radical Damage and its Control. Vol 28 Elsevier Science, Amsterdam.

Sutton HC, Winterbourn CC (1989) On the participation of higher oxidation states of iron and copper in Fenton reactions. *Free Radic. Biol. Med.* 6:53–60.

Suzuki KT, Shiobara Y, Itoh M, Ohmichi M (1998) Selective uptake of selenite by red blood cells. *Analyst* 123:63–67.

Suzuki KT (2005) Metabolomics of selenium: Se metabolites based on speciation studies. *J. Health Sci.* 51:107–114.

Tanaka T, Halicka HD, Huag X, Traganos F, Darzynkiewicz Z (2006) Constitutive histone H2AX phosphorylation and ATM activation, the reporters of DNA damage by endogenous oxidants. *Cell Cycle* 5:1940–1945.

Thorlaksdottir AY, Jonsson JJ, Tryggvadottir L, Skuladottir GV, Petursdottir AL, Ogmundsdottir HM, Eyfjord JE, Hardardottir I (2007) Positive association between DNA strand breaks in peripheral blood mononuclear cells and polyunsaturated fatty acids in red blood cells from women. *Nutr. Cancer* 59:21–28.

Vives Corrons JL, Miguel-Garcia A, Pujades MA, Miguel-Sosa A, Cambiazzo S, Linares M, Dibarrart MT, Calvo MA (1995) Increased susceptibility of microcytic red blood cells to in vitro oxidative stress. *Eur. J. Haematol.* 55:327–331.

Wang J, Pantopoulos K (2011) Regulation of cellular iron metabolism. *Biochem. J.* 434:365–381.

West AR, Oates PS (2008) Mechanisms of heme iron absorption: current questions and controversies. *World J. Gastroenterol.* 14:4101–4110.

Yetgin S, Hincal F, Basaran N, Ciliv G (1992) Serum selenium status in children with iron deficiency anemia. *Acta Haematol.* 88:85–88.

In: Anemia
Editor: Alice Hallman

ISBN: 978-1-63321-775-1
© 2014 Nova Science Publishers, Inc.

Chapter 3

Influence of Iron Deficiency Anaemia on Bone Metabolism

Javier Díaz-Castro[1,2,*], Silvia Hijano[1,2], Mario Pulido-Moran[1,3], Naroa Kajarabille[1,2] and Julio J. Ochoa[1,2]

[1]Institute of Nutrition and Food Technology "José Mataix Verdú". Biomedical Research Center, University of Granada, Granada, Spain
[2]Departament of Physiology, Faculty of Pharmacy, Campus de Cartuja, University of Granada, Granada, Spain
[3]Departament of Biochemistry and Molecular Biology II, Faculty of Pharmacy, Campus de Cartuja, University of Granada, Granada, Spain

Abstract

There is a growing body of evidence from animal research, epidemiologic, and clinical studies indicating an association between osteopenia and anaemia. Fe intake is directly correlated with mineral bone density and Fe deficiency diminishes the mineral bone content, the bone mass and mechanical resistance. There is also an association of

---

[*] Corresponding author: Department of Physiology and Institute of Nutrition and Food Technology, University of Granada, Biomedical Research Centre, Health Sciences Technological Park, Avenida del Conocimiento s/n, Armilla, 18071 Granada, Spain, Tel.: +34 958241000 ext. 20303. E-mail address: javierdc@ugr.es

hemoglobin levels with the cortical bone mineralization and density. Several diseases characterized by low hemoglobin levels or Fe deficiency anemia have been associated with an increased risk of bone loss or osteoporosis. In fact, pernicious anemia is directly correlated with increased risk of osteoporotic fractures. Fe deficieny diminishes bone matrix formation, reducing the amount of procollagen type I N-terminal propeptide released to the sreum under these conditions. Bone resorption process increases in Fe deficiency as shown by the increase of serum parathyroid hormone, tartrate-resistant acid phosphatase and levels of degradation products from C-terminal telopeptides of type I collagen. In addition, mineralization process is also affected by Fe deficiency, because Ca and P content in femur decreases markedly, due to the increase in PTH and cortisol induced by Fe deficiency. Osteoblast function and bone formation are strongly oxygen-dependent. Hypoxic condition (a consequence from decreased oxygen delivery in Fe deficiency anaemia) diminishes bone formation. The inhibitory effects of hypoxia are due to decreased osteoblast proliferation and differentiation. In addition, hypoxia stimulate osteoclast activity in favor of pathological resorption. In conclusion, Fe deficiency anaemia has a significant impact upon bone, affecting bone mineralization, decreasing the matrix formation and increasing bone resorption, therefore it is of great interest to assess bone status in situation of Fe deficiency anaemia.

1. Introduction

1.1. Bone Turnover

Bones is a metabolically active tissue that undergoes continuous remodelling to cope with the body's Ca requirements and to repair microscopic damage in a dynamic process where osteoblasts are responsible for bone formation and osteoclasts for its resorption. These processes rely on the activity of osteoclasts (resorption), osteoblasts (formation) and osteocytes (maintenance). Under normal conditions, bone resorption and formation are tightly coupled to each other, so that the amount of bone removed is always equal to the amount of newly formed bone. The entire skeleton is replaced every 10 years in adults, and around 10% of the skeleton is involved in bone remodelling at any one time. This balance or turnover is achieved and regulated through the action of several hormones (PTH, vitamin D, osteocalcin, alkaline phosphatase...) and local mediators (cytokines, growth factors...). In contrast, growth, ageing, metabolic bone diseases, states of increased or decreased mobility, therapeutic interventions, nutritional deficiencies and many other conditions are characterised by imbalances in bone turnover.

The results of such uncoupling in bone turnover are often changes in bone structure, strength, mineralization and mass (Figure 1).

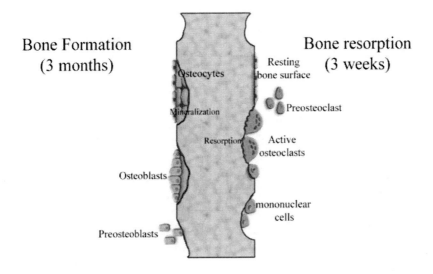

Figure 1. The bone turnover cycle. The resorption (osteoclast) phase takes approximately 3 weeks days, which is then followed by a formation (osteoblast) phase that can last for up to 3 months.

Osteoblasts are specialized mesenchymal cells that undergo a process of maturation where genes like core-binding factor a1 (Cbfa1) and osterix (Osx) play a very important role.

Moreover, it was found recently that the Wnt/b-catenin pathway plays a part on osteoblast differentiation and proliferation. Osteoblasts have also a role in the regulation of bone resorption through receptor activator of nuclear factor-kB (RANK) ligand (RANKL), that links to its receptor, RANK, on the surface of pre-osteoclast cells, inducing their differentiation and fusion. On the other hand, osteoblasts secrete a soluble decoy receptor (osteoprotegerin, OPG) that blocks RANK/RANKL interaction by binding to RANKL and, thus, prevents osteoclast differentiation and activation. Therefore, the balance between RANKL and OPG determines the formation and activity of osteoclasts (Caetano Lopes et al., 2007).

Osteoclasts are the cells that degrade (resorb) bone during normal bone remodeling and in pathologic states in which bone resorption is increased.

Osteoclasts form microscopic trenches on the surfaces of bone trabeculae in the spongy bone by secreting hydrochloric acid and proteases, such as cathepsin K, into an extracellular lyzosomal compartment beneath a ruffled part of their basal cell membrane to dissolve the mineral and matrix components of bone simultaneously.

Precursors of osteoblasts, the cells that form bone, are recruited to these trenches from the adjacent bone marrow stromal cell population and differentiate into osteoblasts, which lay down new matrix and mineralize it (Boyce et al., 2009). Bone remodeling can be increased in response to many influences, including mechanical strain, cytokines, hormones, growth and dietary factors.

A number of nutrients have crucial roles in the development and maturation of bone. Ca in particular has received a great amount of interest because of its impact on the bone disease osteoporosis.

This is a lifelong disease in which peak bone mass in the late teens can lessen the risk of development later in life. Development of osteoporosis is also dependent upon other factors and nutrients, such as vitamin D, estrogen and weight-bearing exercise. Other nutrients that may have an impact on bone physiology include protein, vitamin C, Cu and Fe (Medeiros et al., 2002).

2. Iron Deficiency Anaemia and Bone Turnover

2.1. Iron Deficiency and Bone Mineralization

There is a growing body of evidence from animal research, epidemiologic, and clinical studies indicating an association between osteopenia and anaemia. The relation between Fe and the bone metabolism, has received attention, revealing that Fe intake is directly correlated with the mineral bone density in women postmenopausal women (Harris et al., 2003; Maurer et al., 2005). Several authors (Medeiros y col. (1997, 2002, 2004); Campos et al., 1998; Parelman y col. (2006) y Katsumata y col. (2006;2009) Campos et al., 2007; Diaz-Castro et al., 2012 have demonstrated that Fe deficiency diminishes the mineral bone content, the bone mass and mechanical resistance. Kipp et al. (2002) reported that, when iron-deficient rats were compared with a weight matched control group, cortical and cancellous bone were significantly decreased, supporting an independent effect of iron upon bone morphometry.

Campos et al. (2007) indicated that the anemia produces a high degree of bone demineralization, with a lower Ca and P storage in femur of anaemic rats. After the consumption of a diet with a normal Fe content, Ca and P concentrations increases in sternum, but not in femur, revealing that bone demineralization was kept even after the recovery of the anemia. In addition, when severe Fe deficiency occurs, a feedback effect becomes established, in which the lower degree of metabolism results in less haemoglobin being produced, and thus less oxygen is transported, resulting, in turn, in a lower degree of metabolic reactions. Furthermore, there is an increase in the number of leucocytes and platelets, and also in the concentration of cortisol in serum. This fact is explained by the reduction in the activity of monoaminooxidase (MAO) in Fe deficiency, with a low level of aldehyde oxidase activity. These compensatory mechanisms produce an increase in the levels of circulating catecholamines, which increase the releasing of adrenocorticotrophic hormone, which in turn increases the output of glucocorticoids (Campos et al., 1998). Therefore, Fe deficiency induces hormonal changes, such as an increase in serum levels of PTH and cortisol, indicating an increase in the velocity of bone resorption. In this sense, Diaz-Castro et al. (2012) reported an increase in PTH serum levels in Fe deficient animal models, revaling that this increase contributes to the lower Ca and P deposit in femur of anaemic rats found previously. Moreover, the weakness of the collagen type I fibres lead to a decrease in the mineralization process, because hydroxyapatite crystals might not be deposited properly when the collagen fibres does not bring together the suitable characteristics of rigidity, flexibility and resistance.

In a large Italian cohort with elder subjects (Cesari et al., 2005), they studied the relationship between bone mass and hemoglobin levels in 420 men and 530 postmenopausal women in this cohort (there was 56 anemic females). The authors found that hemoglobin levels and anemia were negatively and independently associated with bone mass and density and they suggested that the bone loss associated with Hb levels occurs mainly in the cortical bone. An explanation for the relationship of anemia and hemoglobin levels with bone density might be provided by a study conducted by Fujimoto et al. (1999), in which, by combining results from animal and human models, they suggested that hypoxemia can affect mineral density and might be a risk factor for bone loss. In fact, the authors showed that patients with low PaO_2 presented a decreased bone mineral density. Furthermore, to exclude the hypothesis that limited exercise was influencing their results, they conducted an animal experiment and showed that a significantly lower bone density was found in hypoxemic rats than in normoxemic rats.

Cesari et al. (2005) have reported a strong association of hemoglobin levels with the cortical bone mineralization and density. Age-related bone remodeling and bone loss occur mainly in the cortical bone that becomes "trabecularized" due to an increased porosity. This might provide an explanation for the particularly strong association between hemoglobin levels and bone density in that site. Cesari et al. (2005) also reported a small but significant difference in trabecular bone density between women with anemia and those with high hemoglobin levels. Several diseases characterized by low hemoglobin levels or Fe deficiency anemia have been associated with an increased risk of bone loss or osteoporosis. In fact, pernicious anemia is directly correlated with increased risk of osteoporotic fractures (Goerss et al. 1992, Easters et al., 1992).

Skeletal manifestations are common in both sickle cell anaemia and thalassaemia. In these conditions, bone marrow hyperplasia leads to widening of the medullary cavity; expansion of the medullary space of the skull in combination with orientation of the trabeculae perpendicular to the cortical surface produces the characteristic 'hair-on-end' appearance. There is also disturbance of bone growth and reduction in both cancellous and cortical bone mass. In sickle cell disease, microcirculatory disturbances and bone infarction may result in episodes of bone pain; other manifestations include the characteristic H-shaped vertebral bodies, caused by infarction of bone in the centre of the vertebral body and the resulting disturbance in bone growth, patchy osteolysis and sclerosis in cancellous bone of long bones, osteonecrosis and osteomyelitis (Compston, 2002). A reduced bone mass associated with low hemoglobin levels has also been reported in hemodialysis patients (Taal et al., 1999). Hens et al. (1990) have shown that, as chronic obstructive pulmonary disease becomes more severe, the prevalence of osteoporotic patients increases (Karadag et al., 2003). Patients with thalassemia, often present skeletal morbidity (Dresner et al., 2000). Moreover, it has also been demonstrated that the degree of bone loss is lower in thalassemic patients receiving more blood transfusions (Orvieto et al., 1992).

Another factor that should be taken into account for the bone affectation during Fe deficiency is the vitamin D. Renal 25-hydroxyvitamin D 1-hydroxylase, which converts 25-hydroxyvitamin D into the active form of vitamin D, is a system that involves a flavoprotein, an iron-sulphur protein, and a cytochrome P-450 (DeLuca, 1976). Therefore, in Fe deficiency anaemia, these Fe-dependent enzymes might become inactive and abnormal metabolism of vitamin D might occur, leading to low bone mineralization (Díaz-Castro et al., 2012).

Fe might act as a toxin to bone cells and contribute to osteoporosis or other bone diseases in people with impaired Fe metabolism and Fe overload. Most typical such cases are in hemochromatosis, hemosiderosis, chronic renal diseases (including renal osteodystrophy) and any case of Fe overload with prolonged and repeated Fe therapy or hemotransfusion. It is not always clear whether the insult to bone comes from iron itself, Fe overload-induced hypovitaminosis C or both (Schnitzler et al., 1994). Conte et al. (1989) compared bone mass density and bone histomorphometric analyses among patients with primary hemochromatosis, alcoholic cirrhosis and controls. Densitometric and histomorphometric results indicated impairment of trabecular bone in both patient groups compared with controls, while cortical impairments were limited only to hemochromatotic patients. Similar findings resulted from the study of osteoporosis in African hemosiderosis patients (Schnitzer et al., 1994).

An important step in the bone formation process is synthesis of type I collagen, which is the major organic component in bone matrix. During collagen synthesis, propeptides are released from both the terminal parts of the procollagen molecule. The noticeably decrease in this bone formation biomarker revealed that anaemic rats had an important bone mineralization impairment induced by Fe deficiency. Fe exerts its influence on bone turnover by affecting type I collagen synthesis and maturation (Medeiros et al., 1997, 2002, 2004). Fe is a cofactor for prolyl and lysyl hydroxylases, enzymes that catalyse an ascorbate-dependent hydroxylation of prolyl and lysyl residues, essential steps prior to crosslinking by lysyl oxidase. Therefore, Fe deficiency diminishes the amount of Fe available, leading to a diminishing in crosslinking of type I collagen which could result in decreased crosslinking activity and, subsequently, weaker collagen fibres (Díaz-Castro el al., 2012).

Bone remodelling is a series of complex processes of bone matrix formation, mineralization, and resorption performed by the bone cells. High amount of tartrate-resistant acid phosphatase (TRACP) is expressed by bone-resorbing osteoclasts and activated macrophages. TRACP 5b is derived from osteoclasts and TRACP 5a from inflammatory macrophages. Osteoclasts secrete TRACP 5b into the blood circulation as an active enzyme that is inactivated and degraded before it is removed from the circulation, with a functional correlation of the TRAP activity in osteocytes with osteocytic osteolysis.

Diaz-Castro et al. (2012) reported that TRACP 5b indicates the number of osteoclasts rather than their activity, therefore the increase in TRAPC 5b found in anaemic animal models indicates an increase in the number of osteoclasts, accelerating the increase of the resorption process.

2.2. Hypoxia and Bone Density

Reduced oxygen to tissues is referred to as hypoxia, and is a consequence from decreased oxygen delivery in Fe deficiency anaemia. In normal body tissues, the partial pressure of oxygen (pO2) varies greatly. The mean pO_2 of bone marrow aspirated from healthy subjects is 51.8-54.9 mm Hg (or 6.8 – 7.2% O_2 v/v) (Harrison et al., 2002). In pathological lesions of osseous tissues, including inflammation, fracture, and tumors, pO_2 is evidently lower (Lartigau et al., 1993).

Low O_2 can alter bone homeostasis, leading to osteolysis. Patients exposed to long-term hypoxic states are at risk for accelerated bone loss. Vascular flow to the lower extremities is directly linked with bone mass density (BMD). A decrease in blood flow to the lower extremities (measured as a decrease in the ankle/arm index) is associated with an increase in the annual rate of bone loss at the hip and calcaneus. Annual bone loss at the calcaneus was increased about 30% in this group of women. Women with increased blood flow to the lower extremities have a higher bone mass at the hip and in the appendicular skeleton. This association is independent of estrogen use, pattern of fat distribution, history of diabetes, ability to walk, and exercising (Vogt et al., 1997)

Furthermore, hypoxia has been determined to be a risk factor for osteoporosis in animal and human models. Previously, several studies have reported on associations between anemia or hemoglobin levels and bone density in selected conditions, such as sickle-cell anemia, chronic inflammatory conditions, or renal failure (Korkmaz et al., 2012).

2.2.1. Hypoxia and Bone Cells

The organic matrix of bone consists of approximately 90% type 1 fibrillar collagen. Collagen is a heterotrimer consisting of two α1 subunits and one α2 subunit; these are synthesized as propeptides that undergo a variety of posttranslational modifications to create mature, fibrillar collagen. The initial modification is the hydroxylation of several proline residues, performed by procollagen prolyl 4 hydroxylase (P4OH), the resultant hydroxyproline residues being essential for stable triple helix formation. Like its HIF-modifying counterparts, P4OH also requires molecular oxygen for enzymatic activity. Further hydroxylations are then performed on by the enzymes procollagen- lysine, 2-oxoglutarate, 5-dioxygenase 1–3 (PLOD1–3), in preparation for secretion into the extracellular space and subsequent cleavage of propeptides which renders the collagen triple helix insoluble, and it spontaneously assembles into fibrils, which are then acted upon by lysyl oxidase (LOX) to create covalent cross-links between adjacent lysine and hydroxylysine residues. This binds the fibrils and provides the tensile strength to the collagen fibers in bone. The PLOD and LOX enzymes are also dependent on molecular oxygen for their activity (Utting et al., 2006).

2.2.1.1. Osteoblasts

Osteoblast function and bone formation are strongly oxygen-dependent. Hypoxic condition diminishes bone formation. The inhibitory effects of hypoxia are due to decreased osteoblast proliferation and differentiation (Park Et al., 2002; Utting et al., 2006). Mineralized bone nodule formation by cultured osteoblasts was strongly inhibited when pO_2 is <5% and almost completely prevented when pO_2 is <1%. Bone formation *in vivo* normally occurs in environments where pO_2 is between 12% and 5% (corresponding to arterial and venous blood, respectively). Thus, atmospheric oxygen levels (i.e., 20% O2) correspond to hyperoxia; our findings indicate additionally that bone formation by osteoblasts in 20% O_2 (which may be considered as hyperoxia) is stimulated by about 50% relative to the physiological 5–12% O_2 range. Hypoxia inhibits the proliferation of immature osteoblast precursors, leading to failure to achieve the 'critical mass' of differentiated cells needed for bone formation *in vitro*. It also prevents the production of mineralized matrix by disrupting collagen formation and alkaline phosphatase activity (Utting et al., 2006). Delayed osteoblastic differentiation associated with hypoxia has been reported elsewhere; this effect has been ascribed to decreased expression and activity of the transcription factors, BMP2 and Runx2 (Salim et al., 2004). In addition, delayed osteoblast differentiation in hypoxia can be attributed to the inhibition of alkaline phosphatase gene expression and protein activity and of osteocalcin gene expression (Utting et al., 2006).

The inhibitory response of osteoblasts to hypoxia is reciprocal with the powerful stimulatory action of hypoxia on osteoclast formation (and thus, bone resorption). It is noteworthy that even in severe, chronic hypoxia (0.2% O_2), mouse or human osteoclast formation is increased 2- to 3- fold compared with 20% O_2 (Arnett et al., 2003; Brandao-Burch et al., 2005).

2.2.1.2. Osteoclasts

Oxygen is both an essential metabolic substrate in numerous enzymatic reactions, including mitochondrial respiration, and a regulatory signal that controls a specific genetic program. An important component of this program is the transcription factor HIF-1α, which is a key-mediator of cellular adaptation to low O_2 tension (hypoxia). A central role for hypoxia and the hypoxia-inducible transcription factor (HIF) is emerging in bone biology. HIF comprises a hypoxia-inducible α subunit and a constitutively expressed β subunit. Under normoxia, HIFα is post-translationally hydroxylated by the prolyl hydroxylase domain (PHD) enzymes, targeting it for proteasomal degradation. A limitation of PHD enzyme activity under hypoxia allows stabilization of HIFα and transactivation of genes involved in processes such as angiogenesis, apoptosis, and metabolic adaptation. Hypoxia and the hypoxia-inducible factor (HIF) transcription factor regulate angiogenic-osteogenic coupling and osteoclast-mediated bone resorption (Knowles et al., 2010).

A major role for HIF in regulation of osteoclast activity it has been also demonstrated. The role of HIF is mediated, at least partially, by ANGPTL4. Angiopoietin-like 4 (ANGPTL4) is a recently identified adipokine, which is predominantly expressed in adipose tissue, liver, lung, kidney, and placenta. Hypoxia-inducible expression has been described in adipocytes, endothelial cells, heart, and articular chondrocytes. ANGPTL4 is overexpressed in critical leg ischemia and in the hypoxic, perinecrotic regions of tumors. An effect of ANGPTL4 to stimulate osteoblast differentiation at low local concentrations and osteoclast activity at higher concentrations might tip bone homeostatic mechanisms in favor of pathological resorption under conditions of severe local hypoxia and/or inflammation. One of the few cytokines to affect osteoclast activity directly, rather than indirectly enhancing resorption via stimulation of osteoclast differentiation, is RANKL (41). ANGPTL4-mediated induction of osteoclast activity could be achieved, albeit with reduced total levels of resorption, in the absence of RANKL. ANGPTL4 is activating distinct intracellular signaling pathways to stimulate osteoclast activity. Given the effects of ANGPTL4 on the osteoblast phenotype, this could represent a mechanism whereby HIF coordinates osteoclastic and osteoblastic components of the osseous niche. If we take into account other effects of ANGPTL4, these results suggest a tripartite role for the adipokine in mechanisms coupling the regulation of bone, fat, and angiogenesis (Knowles et al., 2010).

Conclusion

Fe deficiency diminishes the mineral bone content, the bone mass and mechanical resistance. There is also an association of hemoglobin levels with the cortical bone mineralization and density. In addition, mineralization process is also affected by Fe deficiency, because Ca and P content in femur decreases markedly, due to the increase in PTH and cortisol induced by Fe deficiency. Hypoxic condition (a consequence from decreased oxygen delivery in Fe deficiency anaemia) also diminishes bone formation. In conclusion, Fe deficiency anaemia has a significant impact upon bone, affecting bone mineralization, decreasing the matrix formation and increasing bone resorption, therefore it is of great interest to assess bone status in situation of Fe deficiency anaemia.

References

Arnett TR, Gibbons DC, Utting JC, Orriss IR, Hoebertz A, Rosendaal M, Meghji S (2003) Hypoxia is a major stimulator of osteoclast formation and bone resorption. *J. Cell Physiol.* 196(1):2–8.

Boyce BF, Yao Z, Xing L (2009) Osteoclasts have multiple roles in bone in addition to bone resorption. *Crit. Rev. Eukaryot. Gene. Expr.* 19(3):171–180.

Brandao-Burch A, Utting JC, Orriss IR, Arnett TR (2005) Acidosis inhibits bone formation by osteoblasts in vitro by preventing mineralization. *Calcif. Tissue Int.* 77:167–174.

Caetano-Lopes J, Canhão H, Fonseca JE (2007) Osteoblasts and bone formation. *Acta Reumatol. Port.* 32(2):103–110.

Campos MS, Barrionuevo M, Alférez MJ, Gómez-Ayala AE, Rodríguez-Matas MC, Lopez Aliaga I, Lisbona F (1998) Interactions among iron, calcium, phosphorus and magnesium in nutritionally iron-deficient rats. *Exp. Physiol.* 83(6):771–781.

Campos MS, Barrionuevo M, Alférez MJM, Nestares T, Diaz-Castro J, Ros PB, Ortega E, Lopez-Aliaga I (2007) Consumption of caprine milk improves metabolism of calcium and phosphorus in rats with nutritional ferropenic anaemia. *Int. Dairy J.* 17:412–419.

Cesari M, Pahor M, Lauretani F, Penninx BW, Bartali B, Russo R, Cherubini A, Woodman R, Bandinelli S, Guralnik JM, Ferrucci L (2005) Bone density and hemoglobin levels in older persons: results from the InCHIANTI study. *Osteoporos Int.* 16:691-699.

Compston JE (2002) Bone marrow and bone: a functional unit. *J. Endocrinol.* 173(3):387-394.

Conte D, Caraceni MP, Duriez J, Mandelli C, Corghi E, Cesana M, Ortolani S, Bianchi PA(1989) Bone involvement in primary hemochromatosis and alcoholic cirrhosis. *Am. J. Gastroenterol.* 84:1231-1234.

DeLuca HF (1976) Metabolism of vitamin D: current status. *Am. J. Clin. Nutr.* 29:1258-1270.

Díaz-Castro J, López-Frías MR, Campos MS, López-Frías M, Alférez MJ, Nestares T, Ojeda ML, López-Aliaga I (2012) Severe nutritional iron-deficiency anaemia has a negative effect on some bone turnover biomarkers in rats. *Eur. J. Nutr.* 51(2):241-247.

Dresner Pollack R, Rachmilewitz E, Blumenfeld A, Idelson M, Goldfarb AW (2000) Bone mineral metabolism in adults with beta-thalassemia major and intermedia. *Br. J. Haematol.* 111:902-907.

Eastell R, Vieira NE, Yergey AL, Wahner HW, Silverstein MN, Kumar R, Riggs BL (1992) Pernicious anaemia as a risk factor for osteoporosis. *Clin. Sci.* (Lond) 82:681-685.

Fujimoto H, Fujimoto K, Ueda A, Ohata M (1999) Hypoxemia is a risk factor for bone mass loss. *J. Bone Miner. Metab.* 17:211-216.

Goerss JB, Kim CH, Atkinson EJ, Eastell R, O'Fallon WM, Melton LJ III (1992) Risk of fractures in patients with pernicious anemia. *J. Bone Miner. Res.* 7:573-579.

Harrison JS, Rameshwar P, Chang V, Bandari P (2002) Oxygen saturation in the bone marrow of healthy volunteers. *Blood* 99(1):394.

Hens C, Bohning W (1990) Does COPD affect bone mineral content? Pneumologie 44(1):204-205.

Karadag F, Cildag O, Yurekli Y, Gurgey O (2003) Should COPD patients be routinely evaluated for bone mineral density? *J. Bone Miner. Metab.* 21:242-246.

Katsumata S, Tsuboi R, Uehara M, Suzuki K (2009) Severe iron deficiency decreases both bone formation and bone resorption in rats. *J. Nutr.* 139:238-243.

Katsumata S, Tsuboi R, Uehara M, Suzuki K (2006) Dietary iron deficiency decreases serum osteocalcin concentration and bone mineral density in rats. *Biosci. Biotechnol. Biochem.* 70:2547-2550.

Kipp DE, Beard JL, Lees CJ (2002) Mild iron deficiency results in altered bone mass and histomorphometry in growing female rats. *FASEB J.* 16: A273.

Knowles HJ, Cleton-Jansen AM, Korsching E, Athanasou NA (2010) Hypoxia-inducible factor regulates osteoclast-mediated bone resorption: role of angiopoietin-like 4. *FASEB J.* 24(12):4648–4659.

Korkmaz U, Korkmaz N, Yazici S, Erkan M, Baki AE, Yazici M, Ozhan H, Ataoğlu S (2012) Anemia as a risk factor for low bone mineral density in postmenopausal Turkish women. *Eur. J. Intern. Med.* 23(2):154–158.

Lartigau E, Le Ridant AM, Lambin P, Weeger P, Martin L, Sigal R, Lusinchi A, Luboinski B, Eschwege F, Guichard M (1993) Oxygenation of head and neck tumors. *Cancer* 71(7):2319–2325.

Medeiros DM, Ilich J, Ireton J, Matkovic V, Shiry L, Wildman R (1997) Femurs from rats fed diets deficient in copper or iron have decreased mechanical strength and altered mineral composition. *J. Trace Elem. Exp. Med.* 10:197–203.

Medeiros DM, Plattner A, Jennings D, Stoecker B (2002) Bone morphology, strength and density are compromised in iron-deficient rats and exacerbated by calcium restriction. *J. Nutr.* 132:3135–3141.

Medeiros DM, Stoecker B, Plattner A, Jennings D, Haub M (2004) Iron deficiency negatively affects vertebrae and femurs of rats independently of energy intake and body weight. *J. Nutr.* 34:3061–3067.

Orvieto R, Leichter I, Rachmilewitz EA, Margulies JY (1992) Bone density, mineral content, and cortical index in patients with thalassemia major and the correlation to their bone fractures, blood transfusions, and treatment with desferrioxamine. *Calcif. Tissue Int.* 50:397–399.

Parelman M, Stoecker B, Baker A, Medeiros D (2006) Iron restriction negatively affects bone in female rats and mineralization of hFOB osteoblast cells. *Exp. Biol. Med.* (Maywood) 231:378–386.

Park JH, Park BH, Kim HK, Park TS, Baek HS (2002) Hypoxia decreases Runx2/Cbfa1 expression in human osteoblast-like cells. *Mol. Cell Endocrinol.* 192(1-2):197–203.

Salim A, Nacamuli RP, Morgan EF, Giaccia AJ, Longaker MT (2004) Transient changes in oxygen tension inhibit osteogenic differentiation and Runx2 expression in osteoblasts. *J. Biol. Chem* 279(38):40007–40016.

Schnitzler CM, Macphail AP, Shires R, Schnaid E, Mesquita JM, Robson HJ (1994) Osteoporosis in African hemosiderosis: role of alcohol and iron. *J. Bone Miner. Res* 9:1865–1873.

Taal MW, Masud T, Green D, Cassidy MJD (1999) Risk factors for reduced bone density in hemodialysis patients. *Nephrol. Dial. Transplant.* 14:1922–1928.

Tuderman L, Myllo R, Kivirikko KI (1977) Mechanism of the prolyl hydroxylase reaction. I. Role of co-substrates. *Eur. J. Biochem.* 80:341–348.

Utting JC, Robins SP, Brandao-Burch A, Orriss IR, Behar J, Arnett TR (2006) Hypoxia inhibits the growth, differentiation and bone-forming capacity of rat osteoblasts. *Exp. Cell Res.* 312(10):1693–1702.

Vogt MT, Cauley JA, Kuller LH, Nevitt MC (1997) Bone mineral density and blood flow to the lower extremities: the study of osteoporotic fractures. *J. Bone Miner Res.* 12(2):283–289.

In: Anemia
Editor: Alice Hallman

ISBN: 978-1-63321-775-1
© 2014 Nova Science Publishers, Inc.

Chapter 4

Sickle Cell Anemia: Prevalence, Risk Factors and Management Strategies

*Bruna Miglioranza Scavuzzi[1],
Lucia Helena da Silva Miglioranza[2]
and Isaias Dichi[*3]*

[1]Health Sciences Doctoral Student,
University of Londrina, Londrina, Parana, Brazil
[2]Department of Food Science and Technology,
University of Londrina, Londrina, Parana, Brazil
[3]Departament of Internal Medicine,
University of Londrina, Londrina, Parana, Brazil

Sickle cell anemia (SCA) is a chronic illness and is one of the most common severe monogenic disorders in the world. Organ damage, brain dysfunction and the painful vaso-occlusive crises are serious complications affecting individuals with this disease. It is mostly common among people whose ancestors emigrated from Sub-Saharan Africa, South America, Cuba, Central America, Saudi Arabia, India, and Mediterranean countries such as Turkey, Greece, and Italy. The disease affects millions of people around the world and occurs in about one in every 500 African-American births and one in every 1000 to 1400

---

[*] Corresponding author: E-mail: dichi@sercomtel.com.br.

Hispanic-American births. In many cases, SCA is usually diagnosed with newborn screening. Vaccines, antibiotics, and folic acid supplements are administered, in addition to analgesics. Blood transfusions are a common management strategy, and the only known cure at present is by bone marrow transplant. This work discusses the pathophysiological process, the pharmaceutical and nutritional interventions used as well as specific complications management. Stem-cell transplantation techniques and gene therapy are mentioned. The drugs evaluated in-vitro, and some promising pharmaceuticals are also approached in this review.

1. Introduction

Sickle cell anemia (SCA) is a chronic illness that consists of a family of hereditary hemoglobinopathies caused by mutations in the β-globin chain gene. The mutation affects the hemoglobin (Hb) molecule and causes the discoid-shaped erythrocyte to become abnormally shaped and rigid under stressed conditions. The defected erythrocyte often assumes a sickle-shape when deoxygenated and that altered shape gives the disorder its name. SCA is one of the most common severe monogenic disorders in the world. (Naeim et al., 2008. WHO, 2008). Because of its high prevalence and potentially fatal medical problems, disorders resulting from sickle Hb are of major clinical importance.

2. Pathophysiological Process

Hb S is caused by a mutation at the sixth amino acid position of the β-globin chain of the hemoglobin, resulting in the replacement of the amino acid valine for glutamic acid. (Greer et al., 2004; WHO, Naeim et al., 2008).

The disorder occurs in a heterozygous and homozygous form. In the heterozygous form, there are normal hemoglobin (Hb A) and the variant Hb. In this state, patients usually do not show severe pathologic features and, therefore, are said to have the trait for sickle cell. In the homozygous form, Hb A is not present and the affected people have sickle-cell anemia. (Greer et al., 2004).

There are five major contributors to the pathophysiology of sickle cell anemia: polymerization of Hb S, adhesion of sickle red cells to the endothelium, red cell dehydration, anemia, and nitric oxide effects. (Provan et Gribben, 2005).

The defected erythrocytes have a discoid shape when oxygenated, and when deoxygenated, the cells are induced to become sickle-shaped. Sickle cells are more viscous, rigid and have a decreased elasticity and increased adherence to the endothelium. The altered rheological competence of the cells may lead to endothelial cell damage and ischemia, due to the obstruction of thin vascular structures (Provan et Gribben, 2005). The blockage of small vessels deprives organs and tissues of oxygen, produces periodic episodes of pain, and can damage tissues, vital organs such as the kidneys, lungs and spleen and lead to other serious medical problems. (WHO, 2008).

The continuous sickling and unsickling may cause an irreversible sickling of the erythrocyte, known as irreversible sickled cell (ISC). (Provan et Gribben, 2005). The sickle red cell life span is only about 10 to 15 days, whereas the life span of normal red cells is about 120. Since erythropoiesis cannot compensate fast enough, the shortage of blood cells lead to anemia. (WHO, McCurdy, 1975).

Newborns usually are protected by high concentrations of Hb F in the erythrocytes. With a decrease in the concentrations of Hb F, clinical symptoms of SC anemia are usually manifested 8-10 weeks after birth. (Naeim et al., 2008).

There is a great inter-patient difference in the severity of the disease. The pathologic features include anemia due to hemolysis; hypercellular bone marrow with marked erythroid hyperplasia and left shift; pain (bones, chest and abdomen); recurrent infections (viral, bacterial and atypical organisms) due to asplenia, particularly pneumococcus; priapism; upper airway obstruction; cerebrovascular accidents; stroke; retinopathy; subarachnoid hemorrhage; gallstones; avascular necrosis; hyposthenuria; bone deformities; delayed growth and development; leg ulcers; chronic renal failure; chronic sickle lung. (The Management of Sickle Cell Disease, 2002; Provan et Gribben, 2005; Naeim et al., 2008; WHO, 2008,).

3. Prevalence

The prevalence of Hb S is particularly common among people whose ancestors emigrated from Sub-Saharan Africa. It occurs in a lower frequency in Mediterranean countries, Saudi Arabia, India, South America, Cuba and

Central America. (WHO, 2008; Greer et al., 2004). Figure 1 illustrates the global distribution of hemoglobin disorders, such as SCA.

Studies of DNA suggest that the Hb S gene arose from three independent mutations in tropical Africa (known as Senegal, Benin and Bantu variants) and possibly at least one more mutation in the Eastern Province of Saudi Arabia and Central India (Asian). (Greer et al., 2004).

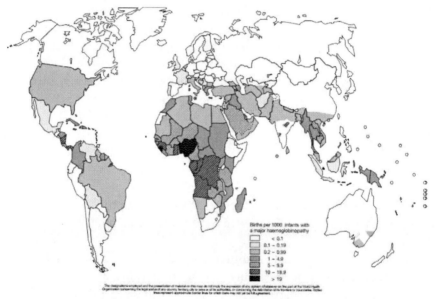

Reproduced, with the permission of the publisher, from Genomic Resource Centre. World Health Organization, 2014 (http://www.who.int/genomics/public/geneticdiseases/en/index2.html#SCA, accessed 14 April 2014)"

Figure 1. Global distribution of hemoglobin disorders, in terms of births of affected infants per 1000 births.

The disease affects millions of people around the world and occurs in about one in every 500 African-American births and one in every 1000 to 1400 Hispanic-American births. In some parts of Africa, up to 45% of the population has the Hb S trait (WHO, 2008; Greer et al., 2004).

There is a higher prevalence of the Hb S in the areas of the world where malaria is more common, and heterozygous sickle cell patients seem to be more resistant to malaria infection than normal people are and that suggests that Hb S is protective against lethal forms of malaria. (Greer et al., 2004; Naeim et al., 2008).

4. Diagnosis

Although sickle cell anemia can be diagnosed anytime during a person's lifespan, it is frequently diagnosed at birth with neonatal screening (NHLBI). The blood sampled is obtained from the umbilical cord or a heel-prick (The Management of Sickle Cell Disease, 2002). The screening is mandatory in many countries, such as the United States of America and Brazil (Government directive MS 822/01). The WHO suggests mandatory newborn screening since early diagnosis and comprehensive care significantly decrease early morbidity and mortality in patients with SCD. (The Management of Sickle Cell Disease, 2002; WHO, 2008).

The diagnosis is based on the detection of S hemoglobin. The main screening techniques used are isoelectric focusing (IEF) and high-performance liquid chromatography (HPLC). Abnormal results should be retested using a different method, usually a complementary electrophoretic technique, HPLC, immunologic tests, or DNA-based assays. The screening methodologies are very sensitive and specific, but extreme prematurity and blood transfusion prior to screening may compromise the test results. (The Management of Sickle Cell Disease, 2002; WHO, 2008).

5. Management Strategies

5.1. Pharmaceutical Approaches

High percentage of fetal hemoglobin and the passive immunity obtained by the mother through the placenta clinically protect the newborns from complications due to SCD. Therefore, prophylactic penicillin therapy can usually begin only after three months of life. (Ramalho, 2002).

The most important intervention in the routine management of children is the use of antibiotics for prevention and treatment of infections. Penicillin or erythromycin-ethyl-succinate prophylaxis are used to prevent pneumococcal infections. Fever is a very common sign of SCD in children and caregivers should be discouraged from giving antipyretics at the first sign of fever since fevers may indicate very dangerous complications such as bacterial infection, acute splenic sequestration and erythroid aplasia. (The Management of Sickle Cell Disease, 2002; WHO, 2008).

Due to the increased risk of bacteremia in children with SCD, immunization with pneumococcal conjugate and pneumococcal polysaccharide vaccines result in a significant decrease in rates of bacteremia, meningitis, and mortality. (The Management of Sickle Cell Disease, 2002; WHO, 2008).

Hydroxyurea modifies disease pathogenesis and is a breakthrough medication for the treatment of SCD that has helped reduce the overall mortality in adult patients. It decreases the incidence of painful crises, and it is effective in the treatment of acute chest syndrome and priapism. The mechanisms by which it exerts their actions are not completely clear, but hydroxyurea is known to increase the levels of fetal hemoglobin. (The Management of Sickle Cell Disease, 2002; Segal, 2008; WHO, 2008).

Iron chelation therapy is necessary when iron overload in patients who receive transfusions regularly. Overload is common and occurs due to the accumulation of exogenous iron when the rate of transfusions exceeds the loss of the nutrient through urine and feces. Iron overload is a dangerous condition that may result in premature death due to iron deposits in vital organs such as the heart and liver, resulting in end organ damage and death from liver cirrhosis or heart disease. (The Management of Sickle Cell Disease, 2002; WHO, 2008; Radha, 2010; Porter, 2013).

Almost all sickle cell patients have painful episodes due to vaso-occlusion by sickled cells and the episodes can last from hours to several days. Medications for mild and moderate pain include nonsteroidal anti-inflammatory drugs (NSAIDs), such as ibuprofen and ketorolac and acetaminophen and opioids, such as codeine. Severe pain, also called sickle cell crisis is a medical emergency and patients will need professional assistance with treatment at the emergency room, day treatment center or hospital. Patients in crisis will receive traditional supportive care measures that include aggressive hydration and pain relief with strong analgesics. (The Management of Sickle Cell Disease, 2002; WHO, 2008).

5.2. Red Blood Cell Transfusion

Red blood cell transfusion reduces the proportion of hemoglobin S and increases the oxygen-carrying capacity. Periodic blood transfusion (PBT) is an essential component of SCD management, as it prevents many complications of the disease, such as stroke and decreases morbidity and mortality of the patients. However, the transfusion therapy is associated with complications to most recipients, such as infection, alloimmunization and iron overload. Transfusion rates are increasing as well as the indications. It is usually indicated for stroke, acute chest syndrome, acute exacerbation of anemia, splenic or hepatic sequestration, and multi-organ failure with severe anemia. (Zakari, 2006; WHO, 2008; Chou, 2013).

5.3. Nutritional Interventions

There is considerable evidence that dietary choices play an important role in the management of SCD. Folate administration, for example, is a prophylactic measure that has become widely accepted in the management of SCD. SC patients commonly have an increased metabolic requirement for folate, and it is usually supplemented at a dose of 1 mg daily. Other nutritional supplements include antioxidants, amino acids and omega-3 fatty acids (Wang, 1999; Aliyu, 2006).

Children with SCD also have decreased height and weight when compared to their peers. Although the exact reasons for poor growth are not established, increased calorie and protein needs and deficiencies in zinc, folic acid, and vitamins A, C, and E are considered to blame (De Franceschi et al., 1997; Williams et al., 1997). Patients with SCD have increased needs for calories and micronutrients, for instance, vitamins and minerals as well as hydration that is important to prevent SCD symptoms.

A diet rich in fruits, vegetables, legumes and whole grains may provide a great proportion of essential nutrients, and appropriate supplementation. Another potential nutritional approach for SCD is a "cocktail" of aged garlic extract, vitamin C, and vitamin E. Significant oxidative stress occurs in SCD and the ascorbic acid role as an antioxidant is recognized (Ohnishi et al., 2000).

Trying to explain the increased needs for calories of SCD patients, Borel et al., 1998, investigated the energy expenditure (EE) and rates of whole-body protein, glucose, and lipid metabolism in 8 African American SCD patients and 6 healthy African American control subjects during the infusion of amino acids, glucose, and lipid. Whole body glucose and lipid kinetics did not differ significantly between the groups. EE increased in SCD patients during exogenous nutrient availability, and the additional energy required for the accelerated rates of whole-body protein breakdown and synthesis made a significant contribution to the increase in EE. These metabolic aberrations may increase the dietary energy and protein requirements of SCD patients.

According to Buchowski et al., 2007, the chronic hemolytic anemia experienced by SCD patients leads to adverse effects on oxygen transport by the blood and to a decrease in oxygen availability for peripheral tissues. Limited tissue oxygen availability has the potential to modify events of intracellular metabolism and, thus, alter lipid homeostasis. They concluded that there is an underlying defect in lipid metabolism associated with SCD best manifested during the fasting state. This abnormality in lipid homeostasis has the potential to alter red blood cell (RBC) membrane fluidity and function in SCD patients. Their investigation was in groups with the same profile of Borel study.

Focusing on micronutrients, Essien et al., 2005 found that the concentrations of ascorbic acid and alpha-tocopherol were significantly depressed, and retinol was slightly reduced in SCD subjects tested. The depletion in the levels of the antioxidant vitamins A, C, and E may account for some of the observed manifestations of SCA, such as increased susceptibility to infection and hemolysis. Vitamin B12 levels are diminished in patients with severe SCD. Patients with low vitamin B12 achieved a significant symptomatic improvement when treated for 12 weeks with weekly 1 mg intramuscular injections. It was concluded that many patients with severe sickle cell disease may suffer from unrecognized vitamin B12 deficiency (Al-Momen, 1995).

Mataratzis et al., 2010, selected scientific articles from Medline and Lilacs databases and evaluated them according to the STROBE recommendations in a review restricted to publications from 1998 to 2008. They used 11 papers, all from the United States of America, being 2 cross-sectional, 4 case-control and 5 cohort studies. In their investigation, they found lower levels of vitamins A, D, B6, folate, calcium and zinc among SCD adolescents and children, characterizing nutritional status adequacy bellow the recommended. The analyzed researches included biochemical and dietetic results.

Patients with SCD that have adequate vitamin B6 and B12 status, but elevated plasma homocysteine levels with suboptimal folate level, may benefit from folate supplementation for a decreased risk of endothelial damage, especially pediatric SCD patients (Van der Dijs et al., 1998; Imaga, 2013).

Westerman et al., 2000, analyzed ascorbate levels of red blood cells and urine of SC anemia patients and verified that ascorbate is present in sickled red blood cell (SRBC), most likely due to ascorbate recycling, despite increased free-radical generation. There was an increased renal excretion, which may contribute to the low plasma levels of ascorbate. The presence of ample ascorbate in sickled red blood cells (SRBCs) and decreased plasma ascorbate suggested that the ascorbate movement across the SRBC membrane is different from normal red blood cell.

The effect of vitamin C on arterial blood pressure, irreversibly sickled cells (ISCs), and osmotic fragility in sickle cell anemic subjects suggested a potential benefit of vitamin C supplementation to SCA subjects. Vitamins A, C, and E supplementation was shown to decrease arterial blood pressure, % irreversibly sickled cells (ISCs), and mean corpuscular hemoglobin concentration (MCHC) but increased hemoglobin (Hb) and packed cell volume (PCV) (Jaja et al. 2000, Jaja et. al., 2005; Imaga, 2013). However, Arruda et al., 2013, found that supplementation with vitamins C and E did not improve anaemia and, surprisingly, increased markers of hemolysis and inflammation in SCA patients. Archer et al., 2008 demonstrated that dietary L-arginine availability could be a possible mechanism for increased nitric oxide production and consequent reduced inflammation.

For SCD, different antisickling agents have various degrees of effect. Antioxidants (scavengers of free radicals) are believed to be major components of these antisickling agents. Thus, it is believed that the higher the antioxidant property of an antisickling agent, the higher its possible antisickling effect, as this enables it to reduce oxidative stress that contributes to sickle cell crisis (Tatum and Chow, 1996).

Amer et al., 2005, showed that exposure of SCD samples to antioxidants, such as N-acetylcysteine, vitamin C and vitamin E, decreased their oxidative stress. These results suggest that antioxidant treatment of patients with SCD reduce oxidative damage to red blood cell (RBC), polymorphonuclear neutrophils (PMN) and platelets, thereby alleviating symptoms associated with their pathology. Additionally, oral magnesium supplementation reportedly reduces the number of dense erythrocytes and improves the erythrocyte membrane transport abnormalities of patients with sickle cell disease (Oladipo et al., 2005).

Furthermore, Daak et al., 2013, investigated whether or not Omega-3 long-chain polyunsaturated fatty acid (omega-3 LCPUFA) supplementation exacerbates oxidative stress in homozygous sickle cell patients aged 2 to 14 years. Their study demonstrated that DHA and EPA supplementation, rather than exacerbating the inherent oxidative stress associated with the disease, seems to provide antioxidant protection. Hence, they recommended providing omega-3 LCPUFA to sickle cell patients to help ameliorate vaso-occlusive and hemolytic crises and membrane fatty acid abnormality.

Recent findings demonstrated that vitamin D deficiency may be associated with incomplete ossification and bone disease, which are well known complications of SCD. According to a review of Hyacinth et al., 2010, patients may also benefit from routine vitamin D and calcium supplements, to reduce the risk of suboptimal peak bone mineral density (BMD) and consequent fragility fractures among other bone complications. There is still the need of setting new dietary requirements for vitamin D, based on recent evidence of increased demand among healthy individuals, and particularly for SCD patients who are likely to have even higher than normal requirement for this vitamin.

Finally, regarding the nutritional requirements, the need for increased fluids should be taken into account. Dietary fluid and sodium intake may influence the risk for vaso-occlusive events in persons with SCA. Fowler et al., 2010, examined the dietary water (mL) and sodium (mg) intake in 21 children and adolescents with SCA (aged from 5 to 18 years) as well as socio-demographic factors. According to their results, median water intake was significantly lower than adequate intake, and median sodium intake was significantly higher than recommended. Socio-demographic factors were not associated with dietary water or sodium intake. The authors suggested that children and adolescents with SCA would benefit from education regarding increasing fluid intake and limiting high sodium foods.

6. Potential Cure

Allogeneic stem cell transplantation (HSCT) from bone marrow has been linked to the cure of SCD since 1983. The need of an HLA-matched sibling donor, myeloablative chemotherapy regimens, the risk of graft-versus-host disease, and high death rates made the risk-benefit ratio unfavorable to transplantation in the past. (Duffy, 2013).

Myeloablative preparative regimens almost limited the application of stem cell transplantation to child recipients, since older patients were too debilitated to undergo the procedures. More recently, non-myeloablative stem cell transplants (NST) with a lower-intensity preparative regimen, has extended the use of transplants to older and more debilitated patients and has reduced death rates significantly. Principles of NST include the lower intensity of preparative regimens and post-transplant induction of tolerance of the immune system. (Barrett, 2000; Duffy, 2013).

Scientific advances are also being made in gene therapy using autologous stem cells. Gene therapy is a promising alternative to HSCT, once it avoids immune complications and the need for a matched donor. (Romero, 2013).

7. Potential New Treatments

Shi et al., 2013, found that tranylcypromine, an FDA approved medication prescribed for patients with major depression, is a promising potential treatment for SCD. The medication inhibits lysine-specific demethylase 1 (LSD1), and according to the researchers, it induces the synthesis of fetal hemoglobin in mice and human red blood cells. Clinical trials are still to be conducted to verify if the fetal hemoglobin induction is reproduced in vivo.

An existing FDA approved drug called regadenoson, currently used for the diagnosis of heart disease, is on Phase II of clinical trials for its potential anti-inflammatory effects on SCD patients. The hypothesis is that regadenoson, an adenosine-like compound, would decrease the severity of the disease by reducing vaso-occlusive crises, pulmonary injury and acute chest syndrome (Jonte, 2013).

Santos et al., 2011, developed a new drug, Lapdesf1, which combines the anti-inflammatory effects of thalidomide and the HbF increasing capacity of hydroxyurea for SCD therapy, and it has shown excellent results in preliminary tests conducted in vitro and mice. The new hybrid drug does not seem to have the toxic effects of the original drugs. In the treated group, there has been an increase of HbF by 100% and a decrease of inflammatory cytokines by more than 70%. The new drug has also shown to be capable of impeding platelet aggregation, which should also reduce the risk of vascular occlusion (Toledo et al., 2013).

Conclusion

Over the last few decades, knowledge on the SCD pathogenesis has accumulated, allowing amelioration of disease severity and a significant decrease in overall mortality through proper and rapid treatment. Early diagnosis through neonatal screening, prophylactic antibiotics and hydroxyurea were responsible for a dramatic increase in life expectancy of sickle cell disease patients. The life expectancy for SCD patients was around 10 years in 1970 and today they are expected to reach at least 50 years of age. (National Heart, Lung and Blood Institute. Reducing the Burden of Sickle Cell Disease, 2011; The New York Times. Sickle cell Anemia: Prognosis, 2013).

Besides the most impacting therapies, supportive measures such as comprehensive care, nutritional approaches and red blood cell transfusion followed by iron chelation have also been important for the management of the disease.

The advances made in the field of stem cell transplantation and gene therapy have also shown promising results for making cure safer and more widely available.

Certainly, more pathophysiological and clinical studies are warranted to propitiate a better management of SCD aiming to improve the quality of life and to achieve even more pronounced decrease in morbidity and mortality in SCD patients.

References

Aliyu, Z. Y. Tumblin, A. R. & Kato, G. J. (2006). Current therapy of sickle cell disease. *Haematologica.*, *91* (1), 7-10.

Al-Momen, A. K. (1995). Diminished vitamin B12 levels in patients with severe sickle cell disease. *Journal of Internal Medicine*, *237* (6), 551-5.

Amer, J. Ghoti, H. Rachmilewitz, E. Koren, A., Levin, C. et al. (2005). Red blood cells, platelets and polymorphonuclear neutrophils of patients with sickle cell disease exhibit oxidative stress that can be ameliorated by antioxidants. *British Journal of Haematology*, *132* (1), 108-13.

Archer, D. R. Stiles, J. K. Newman, G. W. Quarshie, A. Hsu L. L. et al. (2008). C-Reactive Protein and Interleukin-6 are decreased in transgenic sickle cell mice fed a high protein diet. *J. Nutr.*, *138* (6), 1148-52.

Arruda, M. M. Mecabo G. Rodrigues, C. A. et al. (2013). Antioxidant vitamins C and E supplementation increases markers of haemolysis in sickle cell anaemia patients: a randomized, double-blind, placebo-controlled trial. *British Journal of Haematology*, *160*, 688-700.

Barrett, J. & Childs, R. (2000), Non-myeloablative stem cell transplants. *British Journal of Haematology*, *111*, 6–17.

Borel, M. J. Buchowski, M. S. Turner, E. A. et al. (1998). Protein turnover and energy expenditure increase during exogenous nutrient availability in sickle cell disease. *Am J Clin Nutr.*, *68*, 607-14.

Buchowsky, M. S. Swift, L. L. Akohoue, S. A. et al. (2007). Defects in Postabsorptive Plasma Homeostasis of Fatty Acids in Sickle Cell Disease. *J Parenter Enteral Nutr.*, *31*, 263.

Chou, S. T. (2013). Transfusion therapy for sickle cell disease: a balancing act. *Hematology.*, *2013* (1), 439-46.

Daak, A. A. Ghebremeskel, K. Mariniello, K. et al. (2013). Docosahexaenoic and eicosapentaenoic acid supplementation does not exacerbate oxidative stress or intravascular haemolysis in homozygous sickle cell patients. *Prostaglandins, Leukotrienes and Essential Fatty Acids.*, *89*, 305-11.

De Franceschi, L., Bachir, D., Galacteros, F., Tchernia, G., Cynober, T. et al. (1997). Oral magnesium supplements reduce erythrocyte dehydration in patients with sickle cell disease. *J Clin Invest.*, *100* (7), 1847-52.

Duffy, J. A Cure for Sickle Cell. (2013). Accesed: 2014 June 1st. Available from: http://www.hopkinsmedicine.org/news/publications/ hopkins_ medicine_magazine/archives/springsummer_2013/a_cure_for_sickle_cell

Essien, E. U. (1995). Plasma levels of retinol, ascorbic acid and alphatocopherol in sickle cell anaemia. *Central African Journal of Medicine*, *41* (2), 48-50.

Ferraz, M. H. C. & Murao, M. (2007). Laboratorial diagnosis of sickle cell disease in the neonate and after the sixth month of life. *Rev. Bras. Hematol. Hemoter.*, *29* (3), 218-22.

Fowler, K. T., Williams, R., Mitchell, C. O. et al. (2010). Dietary Water and Sodium Intake of Children and Adolescents with Sickle Cell Anemia. *J Pediatr Hematol Oncol*, *32*, 350-3.

Hyacinth, H. I. Gee, B. E. & Hibbert, J. M. (2010). The Role of Nutrition in Sickle Cell Disease. *Nutrition and Metabolic Insights*, *3*, 57-67.

Imaga, N. A. (2013). Phytomedicines and Nutraceuticals: Alternative Therapeutics for Sickle Cell Anemia. *Scientific World Journal.*, 2013, Article ID 269659, 12 pages.

Jaja, S. I.; Kehinde, M. O. Gbenebitse, S. Mojiminyi, F. B. O. & Ogungbemi, A. I. (2000). Effect of vitamin C on arterial blood pressure, irreversible sickled cells and osmotic fragility in sickle cell anemia subjects. *Nigerian Journal of Physiological Sciences*, *16* (1), 14-8.

Jaja, S. I., Aigbe, P. E., Gbenebitse, S. & Temiye, E. O. (2005). Changes in erythrocytes following supplementation with alpha-tocopherol in children suffering from sickle cell anaemia. *The Nigerian Postgraduate Medical Journal*, *12* (2), 110-4.

Jonte, R. New Sickle Cell Anemia Therapy Advances To Phase II Clinical Trials. (2013). Accessed: 2014 June 1st. Available from: http://www.liai.org/pages/New_Sickle_Cell_Anemia_Therapy_Advances _to_Phase_II_Clinical_Trials

Mataratzis, P. S. R. Accioly, E. & Padilha, P. C. (2010). Micronutrient deficiency in children and adolescents with sickle cell anemia: a systematic review. *Rev. Bras. Hematol. Hemoter.*, *32* (3), 247-56.

McCarty, M. F. (2010). Potential utility of full-spectrum antioxidant therapy, citrulline, and dietary nitrate in the management of sickle cell disease. *Medical Hypotheses*, *74*, 1055-8.

McCurdy, P. R. Mahmood, L. & Sherman A. S. (1975). Red cell life span in sickle cell-hemoglobin C disease with a note about sickle cell-hemoglobin O $_{ARAB}$. *Blood*, *45*, 273-9.

Morris C. R. (2008). Mechanisms of vasculopathy in sickle cell disease and thalassemia. *Hematol Am Soc Hematol Educ Program.*, 2008 (1), 177-85.

Naeim, F. Rao, P. N. & Grody, W. W. (2008). Acute myeloid Leukemia. Hematopathology Morphology, Immunophenotype, Cytogenetics, and Molecular Approaches. (1st ed.). Amsterdam, UK: Elsevier.

National Heart, Lung and Blood Institute. Reducing the Burden of Sickle Cell Disease. (2011). Accessed: 2014 June 15th. Available from: http://www.nhlbi.nih.gov/news/spotlight/success/reducing-the-burden-of-sickle-cell-disease.html.

National Heart, Lung and Blood Institute. The Management of Sickle Cell Disease. (2002). Accessed: 2014 May 1ST. Available from: http://www.nhlbi.nih.gov/health/prof/blood/sickle/sc_mngt.pdf.Fourth Edition.

Ohnishi, S. T., Ohnishi, T. & Ogunmola, G. B. (2000). Sickle cell anemia: a potential nutritional approach for a molecular disease. *Nutrition*, *16* (5), 330-8.

Oladipo, O. O. Temiye, E. O. Ezeaka, V. C. & Obamanu, P. (2005). Serum magnesium, phosphate and calcium in Nigerian children with sickle cell disease. *West African Journal of Medicine*, *24* (2), 120-3.

Porter, J. & Garbowski, M. (2013). Consequences and management of iron overload in sickle cell disease. *Hematology*, 2013 (1), 447-56.

Provan, D. & Gribben, J. (2005). Molecular Hematology. (2nd ed.) Boston, MA: Blackwell Publishing.

Raghupathy, R. Manwani, D. & Little, J. A. (2010). Iron Overload in Sickle Cell Disease. *Advances in Hematology*. 2010, Article ID 272940, 9 pages.

Ramalho, A. S. Magna, L. A. & Paiva-e-Silva, R. B. (2002). Government directive MS 822/01 of the Brazilian Ministry of Health and neonatal screening of hemoglobinopathies. *Rev Bras Hematol Hemoter*, *24* (4), 244-50.

Romero, Z. Urbinati, F. Geiger, S. Cooper, A. R.; Wherley, J. et al. (2013). β-globin gene transfer to human bone marrow for sickle cell disease. *J Clin Invest.*, *123* (8), 3317-30.

Santos, JL; Lanaro, C.; Lima, L. M. Gambero,S. Franco-Penteado, C. F. et al. (2011). Design, Synthesis, and Pharmacological Evaluation of Novel Hybrid Compounds to Treat Sickle Cell Disease Symptoms. *J. Med. Chem*, *54* (16), 5811-9.

Segal, J. B., Strouse, J. J., Beach, M. C., Haywood, C., Witkop, C. et al. Hydroxyurea for the Treatment of Sickle Cell Disease. (2008). Accessed: 2014 May 15th. Available from: http://www.ncbi.nlm.nih.gov/books/NBK38499/

Shi, L. Cui, S. Engel, J. D. & Tanabe, O. (2013). Lysine-specific demethylase 1 is a therapeutic target for fetal hemoglobin induction. *Nature Medicine*, *19*, 291-4.

Tatum, V. L. & Chow, C. K. (1996). Antioxidant status and susceptibility of sickle erythrocytes to oxidative and osmotic stress. *Free Radical Research*, *25* (2), 133-9.

The New York Times. Sickle cell Anemia: Prognosis. (2013). Accessed: 2014 June 15th. Available from: http://www.nytimes.com/health/guides/disease/sickle-cell-anemia/prognosis.html.

Toledo, K. Brazilian drug shows good results against sickle cell anemia. (2013). Accessed: 2014 June 2nd. Available from: http://agencia.fapesp.br/en/17846

Tshilolo, L., Kafando, E., Sawadogo, M., Cotton, F., Vertongen, F. et al. (2008). Neonatal screening and clinical care programmes for sickle cell disorders in sub-Saharan Africa: lessons from pilot studies. *Public Health.*, *122* (9), 933-41.

van der Dijs, F. P., Schnog, J. J., Brouwer D. A., Velvis, H. J., van den Berg, G. A. et al. (1998). Elevated homocysteine levels indicate suboptimal folate status in pediatric sickle cell patients. *American Journal of Hematology*, *59* (3) 192-8.

Wang, W. C. (1999). Role of nutritional supplement in sickle cell disease. *J Pediatr Hematol Oncol.*, *21* (3), 176-8.

Westerman, M. P., Zhang, Y., McConnell, J. P., Chezick, P. A., Neelam, R. et al. (2000). Ascorbate levels in red blood cells and urine in patients with sickle cell anemia. *American Journal of Hematology*, *65* (2), 174-5.

Williams, R., George, E. O. & Wang, W. (1997). Nutrition assessment in children with sickle cell disease. *Journal of the Association for Academic Minority Physicians*, *8* (3), 44-48.

World Health Organization. Genes and human disease. (2008). Accessed: 2014 May 5th. Available from: http://www.who.int/genomics/public/geneticdiseases/en/index2.html#SCA.

World Health Organization. Neville, K. A. & Panepinto, J. A. 18th Expert Committee on the Selection and Use of Essential Medicines. Pharmacotherapy of Sickle Cell Disease. (2011). Accessed: 2014 May 6th. Available from: http://www.who.int/selection_medicines/ committees /expert/18/applications/Sicklecell.pdf

In: Anemia
Editor: Alice Hallman

ISBN: 978-1-63321-775-1
© 2014 Nova Science Publishers, Inc.

Chapter 5

Anemia in Myelodysplastic Syndromes

Alicia Enrico, M.D.[1,*]*, María Gabriela Flores, M.D.*[2]*,
Laura Kornblihtt, M.D., Ph.D.*[3]*, Elsa Nucifora, M.D.*[4]*,
Yesica Bestach, M.Sc.*[5]*, Irene B. Larripa, Ph.D.*[5]*,
and Carolina B. Belli, Ph.D.*[5]

[1]Área de Hematología, Hospital Italiano, La Plata, Argentina
[2]Servicio de Hematología, Hospital General de Agudos "C Durand",
Buenos Aires, Argentina
[3]División Hematología, Hospital de Clínicas "J de San Martín",
Universidad de Buenos Aires, Buenos Aires, Argentina
[4]Servicio de Hematología, Hospital Italiano, Buenos Aires, Argentina
[5]Laboratorio de Genética en Hematología, Instituto de Medicina
Experimental (IMEX-CONICET)/ ANM, Academia Nacional
de Medicina, Buenos Aires, Argentina

---

* On behalf of the Argentine MDS Study Group, Argentine Society of Hematology; Buenos Aires, Argentina.
Corresponding Author: Dr. Carolina B. Belli, PhD. Laboratorio de Genética en Hematología, Instituto de Medicina Experimental (IMEX– CONICET)/, Academia Nacional de Medicina (ANM), Pacheco de Melo 3081, CP1425, Buenos Aires, Argentina. Phone Number: 54-11-4805-8803. Fax Number: 54-11-4803-9475. E-mail: cbelli@hematologia.anm.edu.ar.

Abstract

One of the most challenging problems in hematology is the heterogeneous group of disorders that were formally defined as Myelodysplastic Syndromes (MDS) by the French–American–British Cooperative Group in 1982. MDS are clonal disorders of hematopoietic stem cells with a propensity to leukemic evolution. Idiopathic MDS occur mainly in older persons with an incidence of 5 per 100,000 persons per year in the general population that increases to 20 to 50 per year after 60 years of age.

The bone marrow is normo/hiper-cellular, displays various morphologic abnormalities and the stem cells show defective capacity for self-renewal and differentiation leading into an ineffective hematopoiesis. Most patients are initially asymptomatic, and their condition is incidentally discovered on a routine blood test. Approximately 80% of patients manifests with anemia at diagnosis, and this percentage is increased in parallel with the evolution of the disease, being one of the hallmarks. The anemia is frequently macrocytic but refractory to treatment with folate and vitamin B12.

The clinical course of MDS is highly variable, ranging from stable disease over 10 years to death within a few months due to complications associated with their cytopenias or leukemic transformation. Since the development of the Bournemouth index in 1985, various scoring systems have been designed, based on clinical characteristic at presentation, in order to define prognostic subgroups. Anemia is well established as a negative prognostic factor. The International Prognostic Scoring System, the gold standard for risk assessment, has been recently revised (IPSS-R) where new clinical relevant cut-points for hemoglobin level were defined, among other changes. In our series of 578 (324 patients belong to the Argentinean MDS Registry) de novo MDS patients, the degree of anemia shows a good reproducibility and effectiveness to predict clinical outcome. Patients were distributed according to the IPSS-R cut-points for hemoglobin level into: 256 (44%) ≥10 g/dL, 191 (33%) 8-9.9 g/dL and 131 (23%) <8 g/dL, with median survival of 60, 35, and 19 months, and time to leukemic evolution (25% of patients) of 66, 23 and 14 months, respectively ($p<0.001$).

The relationship between severe anemia and poor clinical outcome suggests that anemia initiates or exacerbates functional decline, particularly, involving cardiovascular disease which is one of the most common co-morbidity in MDS patients. Also, there is a high prevalence of patients with transfusion dependence who are prompt to develop secondary iron overload, associated with clinical organ dysfunction, increased risk of cardiac failure, and reduced survival.

The great variability in the outcome of MDS complicates decision-making regarding therapies and prognostic characterization of individual patients is vital prior initiating treatment. The main objective in lower risk patients is improving the quality of life, and in higher risk patients is to extend the survival trying to modify the natural history of the disease. Accordingly, therapies vary from supportive care to intensive chemotherapy and stem cell transplantation.

The degree of anemia is one of the major criterions for diagnosis, prognosis and to proper select type and timing of treatment in MDS patients.

Myelodysplastic Syndrome Overview

One of the most challenging problems in hematology is the heterogeneous group of disorders that have been formally defined as Myelodysplastic Syndromes (MDS). According to the prevailing dogma, MDS are clonal disorders of hematopoietic stem cells with a propensity to evolve to acute myeloid leukemia (AML). They are characterized by the presence of cytopenia(s) in combination with a hypercellular bone marrow (BM) exhibiting dysplasia and ineffective hematopoiesis in, at least, one of myeloid cell lines. [1-4]

MDS may develop *de novo* or secondary to previous toxic exposure to chemotherapeutic agents (topoisomerase-II inhibitors or alkylating agents) and/or radiation therapy. Although MDS are disorders characterized by stepwise genetic progression, the precise mechanisms responsible for the initiation of idiopathic MDS are currently unknown. And, similar to most malignancies, MDS likely arise from a genetically transformed primitive hematopoietic stem cell, while subsequent genetic and epigenetic changes contribute to their development and progression. Immune, cytokine, and stromal responses in the host are important to define the disease phenotype. [2, 4] Pathophysiology of MDS is complex and involves abnormalities in the regulation of cellular proliferation, maturation, and survival. Clonal evolution is associated with increasingly ineffective hematopoiesis, progressive impairment of cellular function and worsening peripheral blood cytopenia(s).

Idiopathic MDS occurs mainly in older persons (median age: 70 years) with an incidence of 5 per 100,000 persons per year in general population that increases to 20 to 50 per 100,000 persons per year after 60 years of age. The gender ratio shows a male predominance. [2-5] The association of MDS with increasing age suggests genetic damage caused by hazardous exposure or inherited susceptibility.

The diagnostic workup of MDS includes morphologic evaluation of peripheral blood, marrow aspirate, and BM biopsy specimens, interpreted in the context of the cytogenetic results and adequate clinical information. Diagnosis of MDS is based on morphological evidence of dysplasia and the information obtained from additional studies such as karyotype, flow cytometry or molecular genetics is complementary. [1-3, 6]

The blood smear frequently shows abnormalities in one or more of the myeloid cell lines: anisopoikilocytosis with macrocytes, hypogranulation and nuclear hyposegmentation (pseudo Pelger-Huet nuclei) in neutrophils, atypical platelets and, sometimes, the presence of blasts. [2-3]

The BM aspirate allows for detailed evaluation of cellular morphology and assessment of percent of blasts. This visual morphological examination is essential to establish the diagnosis. Dyserythropoiesis is manifested principally by alterations in the nucleus including budding, internuclear bridging, and karyorrhexis, multinuclearity, and megaloblastoid changes; cytoplasmic features include ring sideroblasts, vacuolisation and periodic acid-Schiff positivity. Dysgranulopoiesis is characterized primarily by small size, nuclear hypolobulation (pseudo Pelger-Huet) and hypersergmentation, cytoplasmic hypo-granularity. Dismekariopoiesis may be characterized by hypoglobulated micromegakaryocytes , non-lobulated nuclei in megakaryocytes of all sizes and multiple widely-separated nuclei. According to MDS diagnosis criteria, the BM exhibits dysplastic changes in more of 10% of the linage population. [1-3]

The BM biopsy allows for determination of BM cellularity, architecture, fibrosis, small clusters of immature (CD34+) progenitor cells or their abnormal distribution/ localization. [6] The BM is normo-hipercellular in the majority of cases, and is hypocellular according to age (<30% cellular in patients <60 years old, <20% cellularity in patients ≥60 years old) in a minority of cases. [7] The immunohistochemistry-based determination of the percentage of CD34+ progenitor cells is important when the BM smear is contaminated with peripheral blood cells. [6]

Additional studies include analysis of BM cytogenetics. Approximately 50% of patients show abnormal karyotype with a heterogeneous pattern not associated with any particular chromosomal alteration. They are most often characterized by total or partial loss of material from chromosomes 5, 7, 17, 20 or a sex chromosome, as well as a relatively high incidence of genetic gains such as trisomy 8, 19 and 21, while recurrent translocations or other structural abnormalities are less common. [8-9] The presence of recurrently reported cytogenetic abnormality is a co-criterion for a proper diagnosis. [6]

Classification of MDS

The first systematic classification was defined by the French-American-British (FAB) Cooperative Group, based entirely on findings identifiable by cytological analysis of stained smears of peripheral blood and BM aspirate in 1982. [1] Accordingly, the FAB classification, based on morphological criteria, defines five subgroups: refractory anemia (RA), RA with ring sideroblasts (RARS), RA with excess of blasts (RAEB), RAEB in transformation (RAEB-T), and chronic myelomonocytic leukemia (CMML). [1]

Lately, in 2001, the World Health Organization (WHO) proposed a new approach, which was updated in 2008, integrating cytogenetic findings, the type and degree of dysplasia, and decreasing the limit of blast count to 20% for the distinction of AML from MDS. Therefore, this classification established the syndrome 5q- as a separate entity; divided the RAEB subtype into two subgroups (RAEB-1 and RAEB-2 depending on the percentage of blasts), eliminated the RAEB-T category and located patients with CMML among Myelodysplastic/ Myeloproliferative neoplasm. [2-3]

Anemia in MDS

MDS is usually suspected by the presence of cytopenia on a routine analysis of peripheral blood. The presence of a marked and constant cytopenia ($\geq$6 months), in at least one of the following hematopoietic cell lineages: erythroid cells (<11 g/dL), neutrophil granulocytes (<1500 /µL), and platelets (<100,000 /µL), is a diagnostic pre-requisite criterion. [6]

Up to 80% of patients manifest with anemia at diagnosis, and this percentage is increased in parallel with the evolution of the disease, being one of the hallmarks of this disease. Anemia is a major contributor to the symptomatology of MDS, because it is associated with fatigue, weakness, and shortness of breath. Neutropenia and/or thrombocytopenia are less common. The major cause of death in up to 30% of patients is complications related to cytopenias including bleeding, infections or complications related to a high transfusion requirement. [10-11]

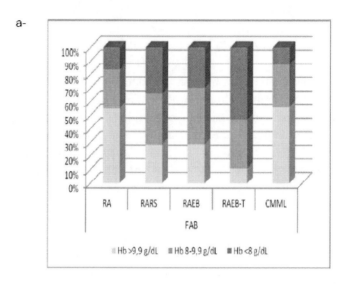

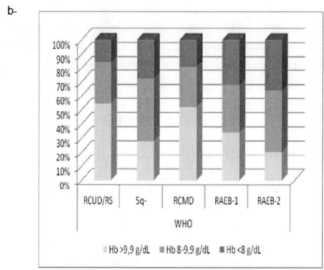

Figure 1. Hemoglobin level according to IPSS-R in relation with (a) FAB subtypes: refractory anemia (RA), RA with ring sideroblasts (RARS), RA with excess of blasts (RAEB), RAEB in Transformation (RAEB-T), and Chronic Myelomonocytic Leukemia (CMML). (b) WHO 2008 subtypes: Refractory Cytopenia with Unilineage Dysplasia with or without Ring Sideroblasts (RCUD/RS), 5q *minus* syndrome, RC with Multilineage Dysplasia (RCMD), RAEB-1, and RAEB-2.

The anemia is frequently macrocytic, but refractory to treatment with folate and vitamin B12, or normocytic (average of the median corpuscular volume: 97.3 fL), and less than 10% present with microcytic anemia. [12] The baseline serum erythropoietin level can be normal or elevated with a wide reported range of 6 to more than 3000 U/mL. [13-14]

In our series of 578 (324 patients belonging to the Argentinean MDS Registry) *de novo* MDS patients, 89% (226/254) of female and 94% (305/324) of male patients showed hemoglobin level below 12 g/dL and 13 g/dL, respectively; 58% (334/578) platelet counts below 150000 /µL, and 51% (297/578) neutrophils counts below 1800 /µL. The percentage of patients that presents with hemoglobin level below 8 g/dL increases from 16% of patients belonging to the RA subtype to 53% in RAEB-T patients which is the more advanced state of the disease according to FAB classification. The same increment is observed according to WHO classification from 16% in patients with refractory cytopenia with unilineage dysplasia with or without ringed sideroblasts (RCUD/-RS) to 36% in RAEB-2 patients (Figure 1). This observation depicts that the severity of the anemia increases in parallel with the progression of the disease.

Physiopathology of the Anemia in MDS

Hematopoiesis is the hierarchical differentiation of multipotent progenitors into mature blood cells of various lineages and functions. Hematopoietic stem cells (HSCs) differentiate into mature lineage restricted blood cells under the influence of a complex network of hematopoietic cytokines, cytokine-mediated transcriptional regulators, and manifold intercellular signaling pathways. The BM microenvironment provides the complex network to tightly regulate the progressive lineage commitment of HSCs. Cytokines are soluble low-molecular-weight proteins that mediate inflammatory responses and regulate hematopoiesis by modulating BM microenvironment. Some are essential for the viability, proliferation and differentiation of HSCs, and a fine balance between the actions of stimulatory/ myelosuppressive factors is required for optimal production of cells of different hematopoietic lineages. [15-17]

The pathophysiology of MDS is a multistep process involving cytogenetic changes, gene mutations, or both, with widespread gene hypermethylation. Even though the driver defects in MDS are not well characterized, the biologic hallmark of the stem cells in MDS is a defective capacity for self-renewal and differentiation. The resulting perturbed interactions between hematopoietic progenitors and marrow stromal cells are probably responsible for ineffective hematopoiesis and may favor the emergence of clones as a secondary phenomenon. The phenotypic diversity of MDS may be the consequence of a dynamic balance among the marrow microenvironment, the intrinsic proliferation capacity of the abnormal clone and the intensity of the immune attack towards the marrow. The ineffective hematopoiesis is accompanied by an extensive apoptotic cellular death of myeloid precursors at the beginning of the disease. And, conversely, an uncontrolled proliferation with decreased apoptosis of progressing abnormal clonal cells occurs in advanced stages upon evolution of MDS into AML. [4, 18]

Molecular mechanisms involved in this aberrant cytokine generation are not known. Immune activation could reflect undesired autoimmune reactions against normal hematopoietic precursor cells as well as effective immune-surveillance against dysplastic clones. Chamuleau et al., 2009, found an activated state of lymphocytes, determined by increased percentages of effector T cells with cytotoxic profile, more skewing of the T-cell receptor Vβ (TCR-Vβ) repertoire, and decreased frequencies of regulatory T cells, when compared MDS patients to healthy donors. These effector T cells with cytotoxic profile express T-helper 1 cytokines, especially TNFα and IFNγ. [19] The over-expression of this pro-inflammatory cytokine is associated with increased apoptotic levels. [15-17, 20] Also, TNFα exerts a negative regulation on the production of endogenous EPO, inhibits *in vitro* erythropoiesis stimulated by EPO or multiple cytokine combinations, and suppresses colony formation. [21-22]

The immunogenetic background may influence the BM microenvironment that cooperates with intrinsic defects of MDS progenitors to increase the severity of certain phenotypic features of the disease. [23] The regulatory and coding regions of cytokine genes are relatively polymorphic including a significant number of single nucleotide polymorphisms (SNPs), some of which are known to modify cytokine activity. According to this hypothesis, we have previously described that the presence of an inherited -308A *TNF*, which is associated with an increased transcription level of this proinflammatory cytokine [24], was associated with more profound cytopenias and the necessity of transfusion requirement. [25] As was previously mentioned, TNFα plays a prominent role inducing intramedullary apoptosis directly and/or indirectly in hematopoietic progenitor cells contributing to the ineffective hematopoiesis, hematopoietic suppression and peripheral cytopenias seen in MDS. [17, 21]

Defective Ribosomal Biogenesis

A second topic that has been described in the last few years is related with a defective ribosomal biogenesis. The 5q- syndrome is characterized by the presence of a del(5q) as the sole karyotypic abnormality, female preponderance, macrocytic anemia, normal to high platelet counts, less than 5% of myeloblasts in the BM, dismegakaryopoiesis with hypolobulated megakaryocytes, long survival with infrequent leukemic transformation. [2-3] The common deleted region in 5q- syndrome has been narrowed to a 1.5 Mb interval encompassing near to 40 genes and the haploinsufficiency of these multiple genes is the relevant genetic consequence of this deletion. [26-27] The decreased expression of these genes, including the ribosomal protein 14 gene (*RPS14*), miR-145, miR-146a and the tumor suppressor gene Secreted Protein Acidic and Rich in Cysteine (*SPARC*), among others, may cooperate to cause several of the key features of the 5q- syndrome and may be related to lenalidomide response in these patients. [28-29]

The *RPS14* is essential for the assembly of 40S ribosomal subunits. A mouse model with haploinsufficiency of *RPS14* shows macrocytic anemia, dysplasia within the erythroid lineage and monolobulated megakaryocytes. [29] Patients with 5q- syndrome have a defect in expression of genes involved in ribosome biogenesis and in the control of translation. Moreover, loss-of-function mutations in *RPS19* and *RPS24*, among others, occur in certain congenital syndromes (e.g., Diamond–Blackfan anemia) that share histologic and clinical features with MDS. [30] The ribosome biogenesis checkpoint most probably results in activation of p53 protein and up-regulation of the p53 pathway in erythroid progenitors resulting in cell cycle arrest and excessive apoptosis. [31] Subclonal mutations in *TP53* gene, possibly promoted by the constant activation of p53, could contribute to progression to higher-risk disease. [32]

Iron Overload

Other important topic is iron overload which is frequently observed in patients with MDS. Iron overload is correlated with serum ferritin and RBC transfusion dependence. [6] However, patients with MDS often show elevated serum ferritin levels at diagnosis, probably caused by increased intestinal iron uptake attributable to ineffective erythropoiesis. [33-34] Other variables correlated with increased ferritin include inflammation, infection, and leukemia cell mass. [35] Some recent data suggest altered hepcidin production may also be important. Hepcidin, a pivotal regulator of iron homeostasis, controls iron uptake in the duodenum as well as iron release from macrophages and is potentially involved in iron distribution to different organs. Patients with an unfavorable type of MDS (RAEB I/II) had higher hepcidin levels than those with a more favorable type (RA/RARS, RS-RCMD), and patients with 5q *minus* syndrome showed intermediate or high levels. In addition, a positive correlation between hepcidin levels and transfusion burden has been described. However, one should be aware that hepcidin dysregulation in MDS patients is complicated and heterogeneous, as described by Santini et al., 2011. [36] On one hand, increased iron stores, due to transfusional overload, stimulate hepcidin production in order to inhibit duodenal iron uptake. On the other hand, there are opposing forces like ineffective erythropoiesis, anemia, and increased erythropoietin levels, which all demand increased iron delivery to the marrow and therefore downregulate hepcidin production. [36-37]

The presence of "ring" sideroblasts is a common morphological change in MDS, they can be found in the different subtypes, and their observation is enhanced by using an electron microscopy which is more sensitive to detect mitochondrial iron overload. Often, but not always, the presence of iron in the mitochondria is accompanied by degenerative changes. Marrow erythroblasts appear as "ring" sideroblasts on Prussian blue staining on light microscopy if their mitochondria contain dense deposits of iron. [38] If BM "ring" sideroblasts exceed 15 percent of erythroblasts in a patient with MDS with less than 5% of blast in BM, the case is usually classified as RARS. [1-3]

It has been speculated that an enzyme defect of the heme synthetic pathway leads to a shortage of heme precursors in sideroblastic anemia which is characterized by abundant protoporphyrin IX, more than ample iron in the mitochondrial matrix, and normal ferrochelatase. Iron, which is imported into mitochondria for heme synthesis, would then lack its reaction partner (protoporphyrin IX) and would therefore accumulate in the mitochondrial matrix. However, such an enzyme defect of protoporphyrin synthesis has been found only in hereditary X-linked sideroblastic anemia, where delta-aminolaevulinic acid synthase, the first enzyme of heme synthesis, is mutated. [39] Recently, recurrent *SF3B1* mutations have been closely associated with the presence of ring sideroblast and they could contribute directly to abnormal iron retention in the mitochondria of erythroid precursors, and thus formation of ringed sideroblasts. [40]

Autophagy in MDS

The evidence for an important role of autophagy in MDS is accumulating. Autophagy is a conserved lysosomal/vacuolar-mediated catabolic cellular pathway for degradation of cytoplasmic constituents as organelles and protein aggregates. Mitochondria are the most abundant organelles to be cleared for the completion of erythropoiesis in order to obtain mature erythrocytes devoid of organelles. Therefore, mitophagy, the selective removal of mitochondria by autophagy, is essential for erythroid development. [41]

BM cells from MDS patients are characterized by increased caspase-dependent apoptosis, [20] reactive oxygen species (ROS) and mitochondrial damage implying possible defects in mitochondrial homeostasis as a consequence of defective mitophagy. [42] Erythroid precursors from lower-risk patients display increased numbers of mitochondria-laden autophagosomes that could indicate intrinsic differentiation defects or could be a response to the higher levels of dysfunctional, iron-saturated mitochondria. [43] On the other hand, this increment may indicate that high levels of functional mitophagy protect these patients from the ROS build-up due to iron-damaged mitochondria until the cells undergo apoptosis from other causes. The genetic alterations affecting autophagy genes in human MDS may be bystander rather than driver mutations, or may contribute to the transformation process driven by other mutations. [42]

Acquired α-Thalassemia

Abnormalities of hemoglobin synthesis are usually inherited but may also arise as a secondary manifestation and the acquisition of alpha-thalassemic clones may be relatively frequent in chronic myeloid disorders, especially MDS. [44] The subset of patients with acquired α-thalassemia shows a median age at diagnosis of 68 years with a strong male preponderance (greater than 6:1 male-female ratio), hypochromic or microcytic red blood cell indices and a median corpuscular volume of 75.2 fL. The development of thalassemia is associated with a worsening of the MDS-associated anemia. Not only does the presence of thalassemia cause additional dyserythropoiesis or hemolysis, a proportion of the hemoglobin produced consists of high-affinity HbH, further reducing the capacity for oxygen delivery. [12]

Minimal criteria for diagnosis acquired α-thalassemia include 3 components: HbH must be demonstrated by electrophoresis, chromatography, or supravital staining; some form of hematologic neoplasia must be present, and the exclusion of any congenital forms of thalassemia predating the hematologic neoplasm. [12]

At least 2 molecular mechanisms for acquired α-thalassemia are now recognized: acquired deletion of the α-globin gene cluster limited to the neoplastic clone, [45] and inactivating somatic mutations of the trans-acting chromatin-associated factor *ATRX*, which cause dramatic downregulation of α-globin gene expression. [46]

Prognostic Considerations

The clinical course of MDS is highly variable, ranging from stable disease over 10 or more years to death within a few months due to cytopenia complications or leukemic transformation. The evaluation of disease risk and overcome of patients with MDS is one of the most critical point due to this impressive clinical heterogeneity. [4, 47-48]

The original FAB [1] classification scheme showed limitations to assess prognosis within the respective morphological groups. Therefore, since the development of the Bournemouth index in 1985, various scoring systems have been designed, based on clinical characteristic at presentation, in order to define prognostic subgroups. [49-53] And, the presence and degree of the anemia is a well-established negative prognostic factor. [49, 52-54] The International Prognostic Scoring System (IPSS), the gold standard for risk assessment, considered among its variables: the percentage of BM blasts, number of cytopenias and three cytogenetic groups of risk. [10, 47] This system has been recently revised (IPSS-R) and new clinical relevant cut-points for hemoglobin level were defined, among other changes. [11] The IPSS-R system showed a good reproducibility, is simple to use since include easy accessible variables, and is expected to be incorporated by most centers until the role of molecular information is better understood in the prognostication of patients with MDS. [55]

In our series, the degree of anemia shows a good reproducibility and effectiveness in predicting clinical outcome. Patients were distributed according to the IPSS-R cut-points for hemoglobin into: 256 (44%) ≥10 g/dL, 191 (33%) 8-9.9 g/dL and 131 (23%) <8 g/dL, with median survival of 60, 35, and 19 months ($p<0.001$), and time to leukemic evolution (25% of patients) of 66, 23 and 14 months, respectively ($p<0.001$) (Figure 2).

Anemia in Myelodysplastic Syndromes

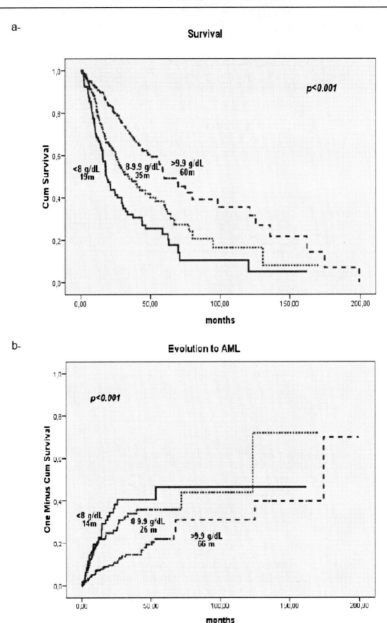

Figure 2. Prognostic relevance of Hemoglobin cut-points proposed by the IPSS-R in the Argentinean cohort of 578 MDS patients. Kaplan–Meier plots for: a- survival, b- progression to acute myeloid leukaemia (AML). Median overall survival or the time to 25 % to AML evolution for each group of risk are shown.

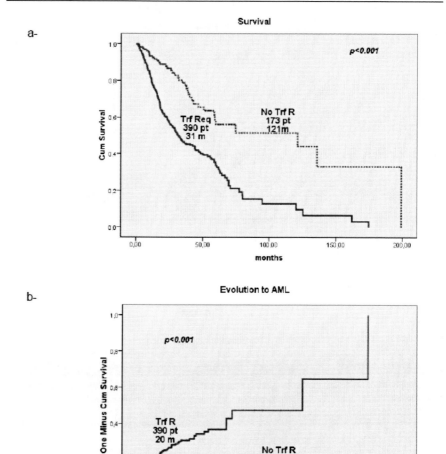

Figure 3. Prognostic relevance of transfusion dependency in the Argentinean cohort of 563 MDS patients. Kaplan–Meier plots for: a- survival, b- progression to acute myeloid leukemia (AML). Number of patients and median overall survival or the time to 25 % to AML evolution for each group are shown.

Also related to the degree of anemia, transfusion dependency has been shown to have a significant effect on survival of patients with MDS. The "red blood cell (RBC)-transfusion-dependence" term is widely-used by hematologists to describe a condition of severe anemia typically arising when erythropoiesis is reduced or inadequate such that a person continuously requires ≥1U RBC-transfusions over a specified interval. The integration of transfusion dependency within the WHO system and cytogenetic findings has produced the so-called WHO classification–based prognostic scoring system (WPSS). The WPSS is a time-dependent regression model and, thus, provides prognostic information from initial evaluation through treatment to follow-up. [51] In our series, 69% (390/563) of patients shows transfusion dependency associated with shorter survival and prompt evolution to AML *(p<0.001)* (Figure 3).

The decision criteria for transfusion of patients with MDS may vary from clinician to clinician, center to center, country to country, and from patient to patient depending not only on their respective hemoglobin level but also on comorbidities and performance status. Therefore, the inclusion of transfusion dependency into a prognostic scoring system has been criticized as being subjective a criterion. [56]

Malcovati et al., 2011, described sex-specific hemoglobin thresholds (lower than 9 g/dL in males and lower than 8 g/dL in females) that showed a significant prognostic value comparable to that of transfusion-dependency. They also recalculated the WPSS risk groups, using sex-specific hemoglobin thresholds instead of transfusion-dependency, and obtained highly concordant risk categories. This modification could provide an objective criterion for prognostic assessment in addition to the WHO criteria and cytogenetic groups of risk. [57]

We also applied the sex-specific hemoglobin thresholds proposed by Malcovati et al., 2011, to our series (males: <9, 9-10.9 and ≥11 g/dL; and females: < 8 g/dL, 8-11.9 and ≥12 g/dL), and this subdivision was useful to stratify patients with different life expectancies *(p<0.001)* (Figure 4).

The relation between severe anemia and poor clinical outcome is well established in MDS suggesting that anemia initiates or exacerbates functional decline, particularly, involving cardiovascular disease which is one of the most common co-morbidity in MDS patients. About 50% of the MDS patients had one or more comorbidities and most frequent are: cardiac, hepatic, renal, and liver comorbidities as well as second tumors. Several groups focused on the description of comorbidities and their potential use as prognostic markers. Comorbidities influence the life expectancy, independent of disease related parameters, primarily in the Low and Intermediate risk groups according to the IPSS. [53, 58] A specific MDS comorbidity score was developed and validated, using the above mentioned parameters, giving double weight to cardiac comorbidities, [59] and this index provides additional prognostic information on patients stratified according to the IPSS-R. [60]

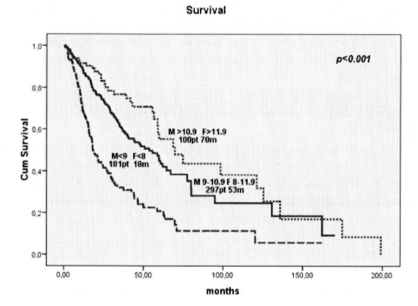

Figure 4. Prognostic relevance of sex-specific hemoglobin thresholds in our cohort of 578 MDS patients. Number of patients and median overall survival for each group are shown.

Also, there is a high prevalence of patients with transfusion requirement that often results in significant clinical consequences. [51] One of the objectives in MDS patients is to prevent transfusion related morbidity and mortality, mostly resulting from iron overload, which may become apparent when the number of red blood cell transfusions exceeds 20–40 and serum ferritin levels exceed 1500–2000 ng/mL. [6] The severity of transfusion requirement, calculated as the number of packed red cell units per month, has been significantly related with cardiac complications. [51] In addition, secondary iron overload determining clinical organ dysfunction and an increased risk of cardiac failure was associated with reduced survival in transfusion dependent MDS patients. [61]

Treatment of MDS

The great variability in the natural history of MDS complicates decision-making regarding therapies and prognostic characterization of individual patients is vital prior initiating treatment. The main objective in lower risk patients is improving the quality of life, and in higher risk patients is to extend the survival trying to modify the natural history of the disease. Accordingly, therapies vary from supportive care to intensive chemotherapy and hematologic stem cell transplantation (HSCT).

Different factors are evaluated in order to offer an individualized therapy for each patient. These factors can be divided into those related to the disease and to patients. The first one involves severity of cytopenias, percentage of BM blasts, and karyotype, among others, that are included in the majority of scoring prognostic systems. [10-11, 49-54] The other main group includes patients' age, comorbidities, performance status and further potential complications. Decision making is complex in this group of patients, with a median age of 70 years old, because ageing is a multidimensional process involving not only physiological changes but also changes in functional, social, emotional and cognitive capacities. All these factors can have a significant impact on the efficacy and tolerability of a potential therapy and therefore have to be exhaustively assessed before deciding on individual treatment regimens. [62]

Although some patients with MDS have clinical problems associated with neutropenia or thrombocytopenia, symptomatic anemia is usually the initial problem that requires intervention. The relationship between severe anemia and poor clinical outcome suggests that anemia initiates or exacerbates functional decline. Also, the quality of life is lower in transfusion-dependent patients with MDS perhaps caused by the fluctuation in hemoglobin levels seen in patients with transfusion requirements and failure to achieve normal hemoglobin levels only by transfusion support. Amelioration of anemia may improve the quality of life in responding patients and can obviate the need for transfusion support diminishing its adverse effect on the natural history of the disease.

The degree of anemia is one of the major criteria for diagnosis, prognosis and to proper select type and timing of treatment in MDS patients. Supportive care and low intensive agents include red blood cell and platelet transfusions, the use of erythropoiesis-stimulating agents (ESAs), or immune-suppressive therapy (ISTs), immunomodulatory drugs (IMDs), prophylaxis and treatment with the use of granulocyte-colonies stimulating factors in neutropenic infections, iron chelating agents, and hypomethylating agents. [63]

High intensive therapies include intensive chemotherapy and HSCT. [63] Currently, the only potentially curative therapy for high-risk MDS patients is allogeneic HSCT. The use of most of them as potential curative approaches might be realistic only in a minority of MDS cases. According to the current data, elderly patients with advanced MDS do not benefit from intensive chemotherapy compared with best supportive care if they show karyotype anomalies, especially those in the high-risk category. [64] Therefore, their goals are focus on prolonging overall and progression-free survival as well as relief of symptoms and improvement of quality of life.

Erythropoiesis-Stimulating Agents (ESAs)

Recombinant human erythropoietin (rhu-EPO) has remained the strength of initial therapy for lower-risk, anemic patients with MDS over the past decade. The doses can be increased from 30.000 to 60.000 UI given 1 to 3 times weekly if there is no response at 8 weeks. [63] Epo may improve hemoglobin level in around 20%-25% of unselected anemic patients with low-risk MDS, with a higher response rate in RA than in RARS, according to FAB, and in RARS than RCMD-RS, according to WHO classification. [65] A minority of selected patients showed a more favorable response profile with considerably higher rates, 40% to 70%. Most of them respond within 6 to 12 weeks with a median duration of response of two years. Interestingly, 70% of relapses are not associated with progression to a higher risk category. [66-70]

The addition of granulocyte-colony stimulating factor (G-CSF) may enhance erythroid response, from 20% to 40%, for those patients refractory to rhu-EPO due to a clear synergistic effect between both drugs. [13, 70] Combination of both drugs showed an erythroid response rate of 39% and median response duration 23 months. Patients with high/intermediate probability of response and with IPSS Low/ Intermediate-1 show frequent and durable responses without adverse effects on outcome. [67, 70] Interestingly, patients with RARS, in which G-CSF has been shown to have the strongest synergistic effect on erythropoiesis, require low G-CSF doses, with a median of only 90 µg/week. [67] Also a response to treatment is associated with an improved quality of life. [68]

Features predictive for response to ESAs include low endogenous EPO concentration (<500 U/mL), low transfusion requirements (<2 U/month), and BM blasts fewer than 10%. [66- 68, 71] Other predictive factors of failure are the presence of an aberrant immunophenotype in myeloid cells or low expression of p-ERK1/2 expression. [72-73]

The long-acting hypersyalated Epo-analogue, darbepoetin, with a longer half-life, seems to be at least as effective as epoetins alpha and beta. Musto et al., 2005, reported an erythroid response rate of 40% in anemic subjects with low-to-intermediate risk. Darbepoetin is administered at intervals of every 1 to 3 weeks as monotherapy or combined with G-CSF and the recommended dose is 150-300 µg/ week. [74]

Kelaidi et al., 2008 analyzed the erythroid response to EPO or darbepoetin and the response rate was 46% in patients with 5q *minus* versus 64% in patients without 5q deletion, and the mean duration of response was 14 months *versus* 25 months, respectively. Therefore, the presence of 5q *minus* is associated with a differential response to EPO. [75]

Immunosuppressive Therapy (ISTs)

As was previously mentioned, one of the important mechanisms in this pathology is an aberrant autoimmune suppression of the hematopoiesis through CD8+ cytotoxic T lymphocytes. Because of the similarity of hypoplastic MDS to severe aplastic anemia, antithymocyte globulin (ATG), has been used occasionally to treat hypoplastic MDS with severe cytopenia. [76]

The use of ATG and cyclosporine (CyA) alone or in combination showed markedly improved response rates in younger (age ≤60 years) and Intermediate-1 risk patients. The recommended dose for ATG is 40 mg/kg/day for 4 days. [77] Other variables linked to response to ISTs are short duration of RBC transfusion requirement (<6 months) and presence of HLADR15. [78] Anemic patients with serum Epo levels >500 should be evaluated to determine whether they have a good probability of responding to IST. [63]

The humanized CD52 antibody Alemtuzumab has been shown to have efficacy in a selected group of patients judged likely to respond to IST based on the presence of HLA-DR15, age and RBC transfusion dependence. Seventy-seven per cent of int-1-risk patients and 57% of int-2 patients responded to Alemtuzumab by three months, even with cytogenetic remission, which was superior to response rates reported with ATG alone. Furthermore, at 12 months follow-up, 56% of responding patients had normal blood counts and 78% of patients were transfusion independent. [79] A rate of 60% of response has been recently reported in a small series of patients with a hypocellular BM, blast count <5 % and belonging to the Intermediate-1 risk. [80]

Immunomodulatory Drugs (IMDs)

Also, IMDs are used as MDS therapy trying to target the altered BM microenvironment based on their anti-angiogenic and cytokine-modulating properties.

Thalidomide is the first IMD investigated in MDS. Daily doses vary from 200 to 1000 mg in multiples trials with either hematologic improvement or partial responses reported in approximately 20% to less than 60% of patients. Responding patients seem to be younger and have RA, thus presenting a similar pattern as responders to ISTs. However, thalidomide tolerance with prolonged administration is poor leading to the creation of structural analogs with enhanced potency and favorable toxicity profiles. [81]

The thalidomide derivative CC5013 (Lenalidomide) is a 4-aminoglutarimide analogue, that lacks the neurotoxicity of thalidomide but displays intrinsic myelosuppressive properties with neutropenia or thrombocytopenia. Lenalidomide is active in a subset of patients with MDS, particularly in patients with 5q31 deletion belonging to low/intermediate- 1 risk, as was first described in the initial MDS-001 study. Among patients with 5q-, 76% reduced need for transfusions and 67% no longer required them. Transfusion independence response to Lenalidomide is achieved rapidly (median time: 4.6 weeks), with a median duration of 2.2 years and some patients now exceeding 5 years. [82] These results have been validated in confirmatory trials (MDS-002, and MDS-003), being actually the first line therapy for patients with 5q *minus* and the dose of Lenalidomide was 10 mg daily or for 21 days every 4 weeks. Also, a phase 2 trial that evaluated Lenalidomide therapy for transfusion-dependent patients with low- or int-1–risk MDS without deletion 5q reported that the overall transfusion response rate was 43%, with 26% of patients achieving transfusion independence sustained for a median of >40 weeks in responders. Variables associated with a higher rate of response in non-5q- patients are lower baseline transfusion requirement, normal platelet count, shorter duration of MDS, and normal serum lactate dehydrogenase. [83] Multivariate analysis of features associated with longer duration of transfusion independence included deletion 5q syndrome, RBC transfusions less than 4 U/ 8 weeks, low-risk IPSS, age younger than 70 years, and good performance status. Also patients that showed partial and complete cytogenetic response had a significant survival advantage. [84] MDS-004 study also showed that higher baseline ferritin level, older age, and higher transfusion burden were associated with an increased risk of AML progression or death under lenalidomide treatment. [85]

Patients with a diagnosis of del(5q) low risk-MDS harboring *TP53* mutation should be considered a distinct group requiring different treatment including clinical trials because these patients are less likely to respond to Lenalidomide as a single agent. [32]

Iron Chelating Agents

Chronic RBC- transfusions are still the main back bone of treatment of anemia and are used as a key therapy to alleviate the symptoms of fatigue, improve patients' quality of life and prolong survival. Each unit of RBC contains 200-250 mg of iron, and as the human body lacks a natural mechanism for excreting excess body iron, chronically transfused patients can became iron overloaded. Patients with MDS can also suffer iron overload from ineffective erythropoiesis and increased iron absorption. Iron overload is associated with an adverse effect of on the morbi-mortality and higher ferritin level prior to HSCT is associated with an increased early mortality. [86]

Iron-chelating agents are desferoxamine, deferasirox (ICL670) or deferiprone (L1), ordered accordingly recommended uses in MDS. Initial studies using desferoxamine in small series of patients showed that its administration diminished blood transfusion requirements and that also was associated with hematological improvements in nearly 60% of patients. [87-88] One of the initial retrospective analysis of MDS patients showed that the use of deferasirox was associated with hematological improvements in 20% of patients. [89-90] Another recent retrospective study, where 70% were chelated adequately mainly with deferasirox or deferasirox following deferoxamine, showed that six or more months of adequate iron chelating therapy was associated with better overall survival and reduced mortality. [91] Further studies, including the ongoing TELESTO controlled trial (deferasidox ClinicalTrials.gov Identifier: NCT00940602), which results are awaited no later than 2015, will more clearly define the role of chelating therapy in MDS, including any effect on specific morbidities or mortality in MDS. It is important to monitor the adherence to iron chelation, potential drug-induced toxicities and the adjustment of doses according to iron status and transfusion needs.

There is some debate over the use of iron chelation therapy because some patients with a poor prognosis may not survival long enough to development iron overload or to benefit from iron chelation therapy. Older patient may be particularly vulnerable to the effect of excess iron and might benefit from early initiation of chelation therapy. Consensus statement provided guidance on the types of patients who are most likely to benefit from chelation therapy: serum ferritin >2000 ng/ mL (without signs of active inflammation or liver disease), transfusion dependent anemia and life expectancy of more than 2 years, except for those patients with organopathy resulting from iron overload, or with planned chemotherapy or HSCT. [92] Guideline developed by National Cancer Center Network (NCCN) in 2013 also recommends chelation therapy in patients with MDS who have received 20-30 units of RBC, particularly in low/ intermediate-1 risk patients and for potential transplant patients. For patients with serum ferritin levels >2500 ng/mL, the aim of treatment is to decrease serum ferritin level to <1000 ng/mL. [63]

Hipomethylantining Agents (HMA)

In MDS, the frequency of hypermethylated genes is higher than that of mutated genes, indicating that epigenetic alterations are an important pathogenic event. The number of hypermethylated CpG islands and levels of gene promoter methylation are correlated with disease severity and survival. [93]

There are 2 available HMA: 5-azacytidine (AzaC) and Decitabine (5-aza-2'-deoxycytidine). Both have been shown to induce *in vitro* and *in vivo* hypomethylation, with subsequent re-expression of pathologically silenced genes. They inhibit DNA methyltransferase activity and, therefore, methylation of new DNA strands. The use of HMA has significantly altered the prospects of patients with higher-risk MDS inducing overall responses in approximately 40%-60%. [94-96] When compared to conventional care regimens, AzaC demonstrated a significant survival advantage and delay in leukemic transformation. [96] As a consequence, HMA are now the first-line treatment for patients with higher-risk MDS not eligible for HSCT. However, prognosis of patients who lose response or progress while on HMA therapy is extremely poor with a median survival after failure of 4.3 or 5.6 months and the estimated 12-month survival rate was 28% or 15% after Decitabine or AzaC, respectively. [97-98] The best predictive model for response to HMA is based on the clinical and biological characteristics of MDS patients: BM blasts, karyotype, performance status, and transfusion dependency. [99]

Regarding the use of HMA in the lower-risk IPSS, there is in fact very little information about their effectiveness. However, the NCCN Guidelines recommends the use of AzaC or Decitabine in lower risk patients with serious cytopenias (particularly clinically severe thrombocytopenia or severe anemia not responding to ESAs). [63] AzaC has been reported to be active in up to 45% of patients. [100] Among running prospective trials, one is evaluating the rol of AzaC (+/- ESAs) in patients with lower risk-MDS, which were RBC-transfusion dependent and resistant to ESAs. They reported a response rate of 30%, being a trend for better response in SF3BA mutated patients. [101] Other trial is evaluating the use of oral AzaC in RBC-transfusion dependent patients with IPSS intermediate-1 and thrombocytopenia, with or without prior ESAs (ClinicalTrials.gov Identifier: NCT01566695).

Conclusion

MDS are a group of highly complex diseases and represent one of the most frequent and serious hematologic diseases that become rather common in elderly. For most individuals, MDS is a chronic illness; however, for others, MDS can be aggressive with prompt leukemic evolution and ultimately fatal within few months.

MDS are defined by abnormal differentiation and maturation of various hematologic cell lineages, genetic instability, and BM failure associated with cytopenia(s), being the anemia one of the hallmarks of the disease. In our series 89% of female and 94% of male patients showed hemoglobin level below 12 g/dL and 13 g/dL at diagnosis, respectively. And, 66% of the overall population present with hemoglobin levels below 10 g/dL. Moreover, IPSS-R cut-points for hemoglobin level and those proposed by Malcovati et al., 2011, shows a good reproducibility and effectiveness to predict clinical outcome in our series, confirming that the severity of the anemia is a negative prognostic factor.

The degree of anemia is not only one of the major criterions for diagnosis and prognosis, but also to proper select type and timing of treatment in MDS patients, being the symptomatic anemia the most frequent initial problem that requires intervention. The relationship between severe anemia and poor clinical outcome suggests that anemia initiates or exacerbates functional decline, particularly, involving cardiovascular disease which is one of the most common co-morbidity in MDS patients. Also, there is a high prevalence of patients with transfusion dependence who are prompt to develop secondary iron overload, associated with clinical organ dysfunction, increased risk of cardiac failure, and reduced survival. In our series, 69% of patients shows transfusion dependency associated with short survival and prompt leukemic evolution.

The great variability in the outcome of MDS complicates decision-making regarding therapies and prognostic characterization of patients is vital prior initiating treatment. The main objective in lower risk patients is improving the quality of life, and in higher risk patients is to extend the survival trying to modify the natural history of the disease. Accordingly, therapies vary from supportive care to intensive chemotherapy and HSCT. The increasing use of HMA in the treatment of higher risk MDS has improved the outcome of patients who used to have very poor survival, but still roughly half of MDS patients will not respond, and the other half will progress while on HMA, or will relapse at variable times after response. The same is true for lower-risk MDS patients who become nonresponsive to ESAs, lenalidomide, or ATG + CSA and need treatment with HMA.

The presence of the anemia is one of the hallmarks of MDS caused by this ineffective erythropoiesis and its management is difficult. We hope that in the near future, with available results from the ongoing trials, we can have more tools to fight against this complex disease.

Acknowledgments

The authors thank the investigators of the Argentinean MDS's Study Group organized by the Argentinean Society of Hematology for the use of MDS Registry database. All authors gave significant contributions to draft the article, critically revise the content of the manuscript, approved the final version to be submitted and declare no conflict of interest.

This work was supported by Argentine grants from the Consejo Nacional de Investigaciones Científicas y Técnicas (CONICET), the Agencia Nacional de Promoción Científica y Tecnológica (ANPCyT), and the Universidad de Buenos Aires.

References

[1] Bennett J, Catovsky D, Daniel M, Galton D, Gralnick H, Sultan C. Proposals for the classification of the myelodysplastic Syndromes. *Br. J. Haematol.* 1982; 51: 189-199.

[2] Jaffe ES, Harris NL, Stein H. et al. (EDs): World Health Organization Classification of Tumours. *Pathology and Genetics of tumours of Haematopoietic and Lymphoid Tissues*. IARC Press: Lyon 2001.

[3] Vardiman J, Thiele J, Arber D. et al. The 2008 revision of the World Health Organization (WHO) classification of myeloid neoplasms and acute leukemia: rationale and important changes. *Blood* 2009; 114: 937-951.

[4] Tefferi A, Vardiman JW. Myelodysplastic syndromes. *N. Engl. J. Med.* 2009; 361: 1872-1885.

[5] Rollison DE, Howlader N, Smith MT. et al. Epidemiology of myelodysplastic syndromes and chronic myeloproliferative disorders in the United States, 2001-2004, using data from the NAACCR and SEER programs. *Blood* 2008; 112: 45-52.

[6] Valent P, Horny HP, Bennett J et al. Definitions and standards in the diagnosis and treatment of the myelodysplastic syndromes: Consensus statements and report from a working conference. *Leuk. Res.* 2007; 31: 727-736.

[7] Vardiman JW. Hematopathological concepts and controversies in the diagnosis and classification of myelodysplastic syndromes. *Hematology Am. Soc. Hematol. Educ. Program* 2006: 199-204.

[8] Belli C, Bengió R, Negri Aranguren P et al. Partial and total monosomal karyotypes in Myelodysplastic Syndromes: comparative prognostic relevance among 421 patients. *Am. J. Hematol.*, 2011; 86: 540-545.

[9] Belli C, Bestach Y, Correa W et al. Prognostic relevance of cytogenetic systems in Myelodysplastic Syndromes. *Leuk. Lymphoma* 2012; 53: 1640-1642.

[10] Greenberg P, Cox C, LeBeau M et al. International International Scoring System for evaluating prognosis in myelodysplastic syndromes. *Blood* 1997; 89: 2079-2088.

[11] Greenberg PL, Tuechler H, Schanz J et al. Revised international prognostic scoring system for myelodysplastic syndromes. *Blood* 2012; 120: 2454-2465.

[12] Steensma DP, Gibbons RJ, Higgs DR. Acquired alpha-thalassemia in association with myelodysplastic syndrome and other hematologic malignancies. *Blood* 2005; 105: 443-452.

[13] Negrin RS, Stein R, Doherty K et al. Maintenance treatment of the anemia of myelodysplastic syndromes with recombinant human granulocyte colony-stimulating factor and erythropoietin: evidence for in vivo synergy. *Blood* 1996; 87: 4076-4081

[14] Ross S, Allen E, Probst C et al. Efficacy and Safety of Erythropoiesis-Stimulating Proteins in Myelodysplastic Syndrome: A Systematic Review and Meta-Analysis. *The Oncologist* 2007; 12: 1264–1273.
[15] Gersuk GM, Beckham C, Loken MR et al. A role for tumor necrosis factor-α, Fas and Fas-Ligand in marrow failure associated with myelodysplastic syndrome. *Br. J. Haematol.* 1998; 103: 176-188.
[16] Marcondes AM, Mhyre AJ, Stirewalt DL et al. Dysregulation of IL-32 in myelodysplastic syndrome and chronic myelomonocytic leukemia modulates apoptosis and impairs NK function. *Proc. Natl. Acad. Sci. USA* 2008; 105: 2865-2870.
[17] Navas T, Zhou L, Estes M et al. Inhibition of p38α MAPK disrupts the pathological loop of proinflammatory factor production in the Myelodysplastic Syndrome bone marrow microenvironment. *Leuk Lymphoma* 2008; 49: 1963-1975.
[18] Albitar M, Manshouri T, Shen Y et al. Myelodysplastic syndrome is not merely "preleukemia". *Blood* 2002; 100: 791-798.
[19] Chamuleau M, Westers T, van Dreunen L et al. Immune mediated autologous cytotoxicity against hematopoietic precursor cells in patients with myelodysplastic syndrome. *Haematologica* 2009; 94: 496-506.
[20] Mundle SD, Reza S, Ali A et al. Correlation of tumor necrosis factor a (TNFa) with high caspase 3-like activity in myelodysplastic syndromes. *Cancer Lett.* 1999; 140: 201-207.
[21] Maciejewski J, Selleri C, Anderson S et al. Fas antigen expression on CD34+ human marrow cells is induced by interferon γ and tumor necrosis factor α and potentiates cytokine-mediated hematopoietic suppression in vitro. *Blood* 1995; 85: 3183-3190.
[22] Rusten L, Jacobsen SE. Tumor Necrosis Factor (TNF)-a Directly Inhibits Human Erythropoiesis In Vitro: Role of p55 and p75 TNF Receptors. *Blood* 1995; 85: 889-996.
[23] Powers M, Nishino H, Luo Y et al. Polymorphisms in TGFß and TNFα are associated with the Myelodysplastic Syndrome Phenotype. *Arch. Pathol. Lab. Med.* 2007; 131: 1789-1793.
[24] Kroeger KM, Carville KS, Abraham LJ. The -308 tumor necrosis factor-alpha promoter polymorphism effects transcription. *Mol. Immunol.* 1997; 34: 391-399.
[25] Belli CB, Bestach Y, Sieza Y et al. The presence of -308A TNFα is associated with anemia and thrombocytopenia in patients with myelodysplastic syndromes. *Blood Cells Mol. Dis.* 2011; 47: 255-258.

[26] Boultwood J; Fidler C; Strickson A et al. Narrowing and genomic annotation of the commonly deleted region of the 5q- syndrome. *Blood* 2002; 99: 4638-4641.
[27] Graubert TA; Payton MA; Shao J; et al. Integrated genomic analysis implicates haploinsufficiency of multiple chromosome 5q31.2 genes in de novo myelodysplastic syndromes pathogenesis. *PLoS One* 2009; 4: e4583.
[28] Pellagatti A, Jädersten M, Forsblom AM et al. Lenalidomide inhibits the malignant clone and up-regulates the SPARC gene mapping to the commonly deleted region in 5q- syndrome patients, *Proc. Natl. Acad. Sci. USA* 2007; 104: 11406-11411.
[29] Pellagatti A, Hellström-Lindberg E, Giagounidis A et al. Haploinsufficiency of RPS14 in 5q- syndrome is associated with deregulation of ribosomal- and translation-related genes, *Br. J. Haematol.* 2008; 142: 57-64.
[30] Quarello P, Garelli E, Brusco A et al. High frequency of ribosomal protein gene deletions in Italian Diamond-Blackfan anemia patients detected by multiplex ligation-dependent probe amplification assay. *Haematologica* 2012; 97: 1813-1817.
[31] Pellagatti A, Marafioti T, Paterson JC et al. Induction of p53 and up-regulation of the p53 pathway in the human 5q- syndrome. *Blood* 2010; 115: 2721-2723.
[32] Jädersten M, Saft L, Smith A et al. TP53 mutations in low-risk myelodysplastic syndromes with del(5q) predict disease progression. *J. Clin. Oncol.* 2011; 29: 1971–1979.
[33] Cortelezzi A, Cattaneo C, Cristiani S et al. Non-transferrin-bound iron in myelodysplastic syndromes: a marker of ineffective erythropoieisis? *Hematol. J.* 2000; 1: 153–158.
[34] Fleming RE, Ponka P. Iron overload in human disease. *N. Engl. J. Med.* 2012; 366: 348-359.
[35] Hershko C, Gale RP. Is iron-chelation therapy useful in persons with myelodysplastic syndrome? *Open J. Blood Dis.* 2011; 1: 3–7.
[36] Santini V, Girelli D, Sanna A et al. Hepcidin levels and their determinants in different types of myelodysplastic syndromes. *PLoS One* 2011; 6: e23109.
[37] Zipperer E, Post JG, Herkert M et al. Serum hepcidin measured with an improved ELISA correlates with parameters of iron metabolism in patients with myelodysplastic syndrome. *Ann. Hematol.* 2013; 92: 1617-1623.

[38] Greenberg P, Young N, Gatterman N. Myelodysplastic Syndromes. *Hematology (Am. Soc. Hematol. Educ. Program)* 2002: 136-61.
[39] Bottomley SS. Sideroblastic anemias. In: Lee GR, Foerster J, Lukens JN, Paraskevas F, Greer JP, Rodgers G, eds. *Wintrobe's Clinical Hematology*. 10th ed. Philadelphia, PA: Lippincott Williams & Wilkins; 1998: 1022-1045.
[40] Papaemmanuil E, Cazzola M, Boultwood J et al. Somatic SF3B1 mutation in myelodysplasia with ring sideroblasts. *N. Engl. J. Med.* 2011; 365: 1384-1395.
[41] Mortensen M, Ferguson DJ, Simon AK. Mitochondrial clearance by autophagy in developing erythrocytes: clearly important, but just how much so? *Cell Cycle* 2010; 9: 1901-1906.
[42] Watson AS, Mortensen M, Simon AK. Autophagy in the pathogenesis of myelodysplastic syndrome and acute myeloid leukemia. *Cell Cycle* 2011; 10: 1719-1725.
[43] Houwerzijl EJ, Pol HW, Blom NR, van der Want JJ, de Wolf JT, Vellenga E. Erythroid precursors from patients with low-risk myelodysplasia demonstrate ultrastructural features of enhanced autophagy of mitochondria. *Leukemia* 2009; 23: 886-891.
[44] Steensma DP, Porcher JC, Hanson CA et al. Prevalence of erythrocyte haemoglobin H inclusions in unselected patients with clonal myeloid disorders. *Br. J. Haematol.* 2007; 139: 439-442.
[45] Steensma DP, Viprakasit V, Hendrick A et al. Deletion of the alpha-globin gene cluster as a cause of acquired alpha-thalassemia in myelodysplastic syndrome. *Blood* 2004; 103: 1518-1520.
[46] Herbaux C, Badens C, Guidez S, Lacoste C, Maboudou P, Rose C. A new ATRX mutation *Hemoglobin* 2012; 36: 581-585.
[47] Belli C, Acevedo S, Bengió R et al. Detection of Risk Groups in Myelodysplastic Syndrome. A multicenter study. *Haematologica* 2002; 87: 9-16.
[48] Malcovati L, Porta MG, Pascutto C et al. Prognostic factors and life expectancy *J. Clin. Oncol.* 2005; 23: 7594-7603.
[49] Mufti GJ, Stevens JR, Oscier DG, Hamblin T, Machin D: Myelodysplastic syndromes: a scoring system with prognostic significance. *Br. J. Hae*matol. 1985; 59: 425-433.
[50] Sanz G, Sanz M, Vallespi T et al. Two regression models and a scoring system for predicting survival and planning treatment in myelodysplastic syndromes: a multivariate analysis of prognostic factors in 370 patients. *Blood* 1989; 74: 395-408.

[51] Malcovati L, Germing U, Kuendgen A et al. Time-Dependent Prognostic Scoring System for predicting survival and leukemic evolution in Myelodysplastic Syndromes. *J. Clin. Oncol.* 2007; 25: 3503-3510.
[52] Kantarjian H, O'Brien S, Ravandi F et al. Proposal for a New Risk Model in Myelodysplastic Syndrome that accounts for events not considered in the original International Prognostic Scoring System. *Cancer* 2008; 113: 1351–1361.
[53] Germing U, Kündgen A. Prognostic scoring systems in MDS. *Leuk. Res.* 2012; 36: 1463-1469.
[54] Goasguen J, Garand R, Bizet M et al. Prognostic factors of myelodysplastic syndromes. A simplified 3-D scoring system. *Leuk. Res.* 1990; 14: 255-262.
[55] Belli CB, Bestach Y, Giunta M et al. Application of the revised International Prognostic Scoring System for myelodysplastic syndromes *Ann. Hematol.* 2014; 93: 705-707.
[56] Bowen D, Fenaux P, Hellstrom-Lindberg E, de Witte T. Time-Dependent Prognostic Scoring System for Myelodysplastic Syndromes has significant limitations that may influence its reproducibility and practical application. *J. Clin. Oncol.* 2008; 26: 1180.
[57] Malcovati L, Della Porta MG, Strupp C et al. Impact of the degree of anemia on the outcome of patients with myelodysplastic syndrome and its integration into the WHO classification-based Prognostic Scoring System (WPSS). *Haematologica* 2011; 96: 1433-1440.
[58] Zipperer E, Pelz D, Nachtkamp K et al. The hematopoietic stem cell transplantation comorbidity index is of prognostic relevance for patients with myelodysplastic syndrome. *Haematologica* 2009; 94: 729-732.
[59] Della Porta MG, Malcovati L, Strupp C et al. Risk stratification based on both disease status and extra-hematologic comorbidities in patients with myelodysplastic syndrome. *Haematologica* 2011; 96: 441–449.
[60] Zipperer E, Tanha N, Strupp C et al. The myelodysplastic syndrome *Haematologica* 2014; 99: e31-32.
[61] Dreyfus F. The deleterious effects of iron overload in patients with myelodysplastic syndromes. *Blood Rev.* 2008; S2: S29-34.
[62] Stauder R. The challenge of individualised risk assessment and therapy planning in elderly high-risk myelodysplastic syndromes (MDS) patients. *Ann. Hematol.* 2012; 91: 1333-1343.
[63] Greenberg PL, Attar E, Bennett JM et al. Myelodysplastic syndromes: clinical practice guidelines in oncology. *J. Natl. Compr. Canc. Netw.* 2013; 11: 838-874.

[64] Knipp S, Hildebrand B, Kündgen A et al. Intensive chemotherapy is not recommended for patients aged >60 years who have myelodysplastic syndromes or acute myeloid leukemia with high-risk karyotypes. *Cancer* 2007; 110: 345-52.
[65] Howe R, Porwit-MacDonald A, Wanat R, Tehranchi R, Hellstrom-Lindberg E. The WHO classification does make a difference. *Blood* 2004; 103: 3265-3270.
[66] Hellstrom-Lindberg E, Negrin R, Stein R et al. Erythroid response to treatment with G-CSF plus erythropoietin for the anaemia of patients with myelodysplastic syndromes: proposal for a predictive model. *Br. J. Hematol.* 1997; 99: 344-351.
[67] Jädersten M, Montgomery SM, Dybedal I, Porwit-MacDonald A, Hellström-Lindberg E. Long-term outcome of treatment of anemia in MDS with erythropoietin and G-CSF. *Blood* 2005; 106: 803-811.
[68] Hellstrom-Lindberg E, Gulbrandsen N, Lindberg G et al. A validated decision model for treating the anaemia of myelodysplastic syndromes with erythropoietin + granulocyte colony-stimulating factor: significant effects on quality of life. *Br. J. Haematol.* 2003; 120: 1037-1046.
[69] Balleari E, Rossi E, Clavio M et al. Erythropoietin plus granulocyte colony-stimulating factor is better than erythropoietin alone to treat anemia in low-risk myelodysplastic syndromes: results from a randomized single-centre study. *Ann. Hematol.* 2006; 85: 174-180.
[70] Park S, Grabar S, Kelaidi C et al. For the Groupe Francophone des myelodysplasies (GFM). Has treatment with EPO +/− G-CSF an impact on progression to AML and survival in low/int-1-risk MDS? A comparison between French-EPO patients and the IMRAW database. *Leuk. Res.* 2007; 31: S113.
[71] Italian Cooperative Study Group for rHuEpo in Myelodysplastic Syndromes et al. A randomized double-blind placebo-controlled study with subcutaneous recombinant human erythropoietin in patients with low-risk myelodysplastic syndromes. *Br. J. Haematol.* 1998; 103: 1070-1074.
[72] Westers TM, Alhan C, Chamuleau ME et al. Aberrant immunophenotype of blasts in myelodysplastic syndromes is a clinically relevant biomarker in predicting response to growth factor treatment. *Blood* 2010; 115: 1779-1784.
[73] Frisan E, Pawlikowska P, Pierre-Eugène C et al. p-ERK1/2 is a predictive factor of response *Haematologica* 2010; 95: 1964-1968.

[74] Musto P, Lanza F, Balleari E et al. Darbepoetin alpha for the treatment of anaemia in low-intermediate risk myelodysplastic syndromes. *Br. J. Haematol.* 2005; 128: 204- 209.

[75] Kelaidi C, Park S, Brechignac S et al. Treatment of myelodysplastic syndromes *Leuk. Res.* 2008; 32: 1049-1053.

[76] Molldrem J, Jiang Y, Stetler-Stevenson M, Mavroudis D, Hensel N, Barrett J. Haematological response of patients with myelodysplastic syndrome to antithymocyte globulin is associated with a loss of lymphocyte-mediated inhibition of CFU-GM and alterations in T-cell receptor Vbeta profiles. *Br. J. Haematol.* 1998; 102: 1314-1322.

[77] Santini V, Alessandrino PE, Angelucci E et al. Clinical management *Leuk. Res.* 2010; 34: 1576-1588.

[78] Sloand EM, Wu CO, Greenberg P et al. Factors affecting response and survival in patients with myelodysplasia treated with immunosuppressive therapy. *J. Clin. Oncol.* 2008; 26: 2505-2511.

[79] Sloand EM, Olnes MJ, Shenoy A et al. Alemtuzumab treatment of intermediate-1 myelodysplasia patients is associated with sustained improvement in blood counts and cytogenetic remissions. *J. Clin. Oncol.* 2010; 28: 5166–5173.

[80] Neukirchen J, Platzbecker U, Sockel K, Tsamaloukas A, Haas R, Germing U. Real life experience with alemtuzumab treatment *Ann. Hematol.* 2014; 93: 65-69.

[81] Bartlett J, Dredge K, Dalgleish A. The evolution of thalidomide and its IMiD derivatives as anticancer agents. *Nat. Rev. Cancer* 2004; 4: 314-322.

[82] List A, Kurtin S, Roe D et al. Efficacy of lenalidomide in myelodysplastic syndromes. *N. Engl. J. Med.* 2005; 352: 549–557.

[83] Raza A, Reeves JA, Feldman EJ et al. Phase 2 study of lenalidomide in transfusion *Blood* 2008; 111: 86-93.

[84] List A, Wride K, Dewald G et al. Cytogenetic response to lenalidomide is associated with improved survival in patients with chromosome 5q deletion. *Leuk. Res.* 2007; 31: S38.

[85] Fenaux P, Giagounidis A, Selleslag D et al. A randomized phase 3 study of lenalidomide versus placebo in RBC transfusion-dependent patients with Low-/Intermediate-1-risk myelodysplastic syndromes with del5q. *Blood* 2011; 118: 3765-3776.

[86] Platzbecker U, Ades L. Clinical management of patients with Myelodysplastic Syndromes. *Hematology Education* 2014; 8: 243-250.

[87] Jensen PD, Jensen IM, Ellegard J. Desferrioxamine treatment reduces blood transfusion requirements in patients with Myelodysplastic Syndromes. *Br. J. Hematol.* 1992; 80: 121-124.
[88] Jensen PD, Heickendorff L, Pedersen B et al. The effect of iron *Br. J. Haematol.* 1996; 94: 288-299.
[89] Jabbour E, Garcia-Manero G, Taher A, Kantarjian HM. Managing iron *Oncologist* 2009; 14: 489-496.
[90] Gattermann N, Finelli C, Della Porta M et al. Hematologic responses to deferasirox therapy *Haematologica* 2012; 97: 1364-1371.
[91] Delforge M, Selleslag D, Beguin Y et al. Adequate iron chelation therapy for at least six months improves survival in transfusion-dependent patients with lower risk myelodysplastic syndromes. *Leuk. Res.* 2014; 38: 557-563.
[92] Valent P, Krieger O, Stauder R et al. Iron overload in myelodysplastic syndromes (MDS) - diagnosis, management, and response criteria: a proposal of the Austrian MDS platform. *Eur. J. Clin. Invest.* 2008; 38: 143-149.
[93] Shen L, Kantarjian H, Guo Y et al. DNA methylation predicts survival and response to therapy in patients with myelodysplastic syndromes. *J. Clin. Oncol.* 2010; 28: 605-613.
[94] Kantarjian H, Issa JP, Rosenfeld CS et al. Decitabine improves patient outcomes in myelodysplastic syndromes: results of a phase III randomized study. *Cancer* 2006; 106: 1794-1803.
[95] Silverman LR, Demakos EP, Peterson BL et al. Randomized controlled trial of azacitidine in patients with the myelodysplastic syndrome: a study of the cancer and leukemia group B. *J. Clin. Oncol.* 2002; 20: 2429-2440.
[96] Fenaux P, Mufti GJ, Hellstrom-Lindberg E et al. (2009) Efficacy of azacitidine compared with that of conventional care regimens in the treatment of higher-risk myelodysplastic syndromes: a randomised, open-label, phase III study. *Lancet Oncol.* 2009; 10: 223-232.
[97] Jabbour E, Garcia-Manero G, Batty N et al. Outcome of patients with myelodysplastic syndrome after failure of decitabine therapy. *Cancer* 2010; 116: 3830-3834.
[98] Prébet T, Gore SD, Esterni B et al. Outcome of high-risk myelodysplastic syndrome after azacitidine treatment failure. *J. Clin. Oncol.* 2011; 29: 3322-3327.

[99] Itzykson R, Thépot S, Quesnel B et al. Prognostic factors for response and overall survival in 282 patients with higher-risk myelodysplastic syndromes treated with azacitidine. *Blood* 2011; 117: 403-411.

[100] Musto P, Maurillo L, Spagnoli A et al. Azacitidine for the treatment *Cancer* 2010; 116: 1485-1494.

[101] Thepot S, Ben Abdelali R, Chevret S et al. Prognostic Factors Of Response and Survival To Azacitidine (AZA) +/- EPO In RBC Transfusion Dependent (TD) IPSS Low and Int-1 (LR) MDS Resistant To EPO, With Particular Emphasis Of Genetic Lesions: A Study By The GFM. *Blood* 2013; 122: 658.

In: Anemia
Editor: Alice Hallman

ISBN: 978-1-63321-775-1
© 2014 Nova Science Publishers, Inc.

Chapter 6

Transfusion in Chronic Anaemia

*Philip Crispin**
Haematologist, Canberra Hospital,
Australian National University Medical School,
Australian Red Cross Blood Service, Australia

Abstract

For the practicing haematologist, one of the most common transfusion decisions is in the chronically anaemic patient. There are unique aspects to this decision in sickle cell disease, where a body of evidence has developed around preventing complications of the underlying disease. In children, where chronic anaemia may lead to developmental concerns, transfusion goals may be formulated to prevent long term complications. In adults, chronic anaemia is most frequently seen in haematological malignancies and myelodysplasia, with the prevalence increasing with age. Transfusion decisions are therefore complicated by comorbid conditions of aging, such as cardiovascular and respiratory illness.

There is consensus in many published guidelines that transfusion is usually appropriate when the haemoglobin is less than 60-70g/L, and generally not indicated when the haemoglobin is more than 100g/L. This is despite evidence that there is a continuum of improvement in quality of life as the haemoglobin increases above these levels with the use of

---

*Lecturer, Australian National University Medical School; Honorary Clinical Fellow.

erythropoietin in myelodysplasia, cancer therapy and renal disease. Even with haemoglobins within the normal range, performance in trained athletes improves as the haemoglobin rises, either induced by erythropoietin or transfusion.

Patients usually are not aiming to achieve the levels of performance required in athletes. They may well cope with lower haemoglobin levels, and the weight of opinion supports this. However, there are no good laboratory measures to indicate when a low haemoglobin might be impairing function and considerable variability in practice, suggesting that the management of chronically anaemic patients is not optimal. This review will summarise the evidence guiding transfusion for relief of symptoms of anaemia in the chronic setting.

Introduction

Chronic anaemia is one of the most common causes of disability worldwide, with most related to nutritional iron deficiency, excess iron loss due to bleeding or both[1]. Haemoglobinopathies, malaria and chronic renal disease are also common causes internationally. Fortunately, for a large number of people with anaemia, pharmacological, dietary or surgical treatment is adequate treatment, without the need for transfusion. For a significant number of people, particularly with primary bone marrow failure, transfusion is the mainstay of therapy for anaemia.

Despite the frequency of anaemia, and the use of transfusion as a therapy for more than 100 years[2], there is a high degree of variability in the use of transfusions. Although there is a fair consensus among guidelines regarding approximate limits below which transfusions are likely to be indicated, they contain a large amount of variability for what constitutes an appropriate transfusion, with considerable flexibility for variation based on clinical factors accounted for within recommendations. Guidelines offer little practical advice on how to determine the appropriate haemoglobin threshold for an individual within the broad ranges considered appropriate[3-6].

In the acute setting, restrictive practices are now universally recommended, based on emerging evidence over the last 15 years indicating a lack of benefit, and even harm from, more liberal approaches to transfusion[7-9]. While these studies provide reassurance that a restrictive strategy may well be safe in the chronic setting, the goals of therapy are clearly different in the acutely ill or perioperative setting than for those with chronic anaemia.

The goals of chronic transfusion therapy vary between the conditions being treated. For sickle cell disease, transfusion aims to improve symptoms of anaemia, and decrease sickling by increasing the relative proportion of HbA. Evidence based guidelines recommend transfusions to prevent recurrent sickling causing stroke in children at high risk [10].

There is also a consensus amongst guidelines for the treatment of thalassaemia on the initiation and goals of transfusion therapy [11, 12]. Initiation takes into account not only the initial haemoglobin concentration in the steady state, but also demonstrable complications arising from anaemia, such as growth retardation, skeletal changes secondary to increased erythropoiesis, extra-medullary haemopoiesis, pulmonary hypertension, failure to thrive and impaired quality of life. Some of these factors are unique to the developing child, whereas others may occur at any age. There is no doubt that the development of chronic transfusion therapy for thalassaemia was the first major breakthrough in treating this condition. However, transfusion brings with it its own complications, and in the developed world transfusion related iron overload is the leading cause of death. Prior to chelating therapy, life expectancy for patients with thalassaemia major were less than 20 years, with cardiac, hepatic and infectious complications of iron overload major causes of mortality[13, 14]. Current guidelines are mindful of the effect of iron overload in recommending a restrictive path to transfusion, waiting to see clinically significant effects of anaemia before a program is initiated. Once started however, transfusions are generally given to maintain haemoglobin readings over 90-100g/L with the aim of restricting complications from excessive erythropoiesis.

The goals of transfusion in adults with chronic anaemia secondary to bone marrow failure syndromes are also to prevent harm secondary to anaemia and to maximise quality of life. If these goals are not being met, transfusion is only exposing recipients to potential harm. A rational, scientific approach to transfusion therefore requires an understanding of how transfusion may reduce, or increase, adverse events, and the impact on performance and quality of life. Although lessons from studies in congenital anaemia may provide guidance into adulthood, there are additional unique considerations, especially when considering comorbidities and competing risks in the older population.

Guidelines in Chronic Anaemia

A number of guidelines have been published, summarising the body of evidence and offering clinical advice on when to transfuse[3-6, 15]. These are heavily influenced by a number of clinical trials in the acute inpatient setting, most restricted to stable, non-bleeding patients. These trials are important as they validate the safety of restrictive transfusion strategies. In the acute setting, where anaemia is correctable, the outcomes evaluated in these studies are highly relevant. Mortality, hospital and intensive care length of stay, sepsis and cardiovascular complications are excellent outcomes to measure, and whilst many of these are also applicable to the chronically transfused patient, no large randomised studies have specifically addressed the effect of transfusion on symptoms or quality of life in chronically anaemic patients.

Most guidelines either avoid the issue of chronic transfusion or provide expert opinion that the decision to transfuse should be based on physician assessment of symptoms and signs of anaemia. Haemoglobin levels are provided for general guidance, usually in the range of 70-100g/L. For the treating clinician there may be difficulty determining when to transfuse, within this wide range of haemoglobin values, in patients with comorbidities and a variety of symptoms. In the setting of comorbidities, symptoms may or may not be due to anaemia and a trial of transfusion may be warranted. The there is a further difficulty in attempting to assess response to those transfusions, with little guidance on how this should be assessed or potentially measured.

In determining an appropriate level at which to transfuse, a clinician would ideally know at what level anaemia may become harmful, information which may be determined generally from large population studies. Furthermore, knowledge that transfusion improves outcomes would be ideal background to inform clinicians in transfusion decisions. Whilst some indication has come from cohort studies, strong evidence of therapeutic benefit is usually provided by randomised controlled trials, studies unfortunately lacking in medical patients with chronic anaemia. The final piece of vital information in assessing the indication for transfusion is the impact of transfusion on the recipient's quality of life and in the absence of proven benefit from transfusion at a particular haemoglobin threshold, this frequently serves the basis for transfusion decisions. In the remainder of this paper, the body of evidence for each of these factors that may underpin a decision to transfuse will be reviewed.

Complications of Anaemia

Anaemia is an established risk factor for adverse clinical outcomes in a variety of clinical settings. In acute coronary syndrome, retrospective and prospective cohort studies have consistently shown that anaemia is a risk factor for mortality and progressive heart failure[16, 17]. In congestive cardiac failure anaemia also is independently associated with an increased risk of mortality in prospective cohort studies. This association appears strong and consistent across studies[18-22]. The level of the haemoglobin concentration appears to have an effect on mortality even within the normal range, with any haemoglobin level below 150-160g/L potentially increasing the risk of death. In congestive cardiac failure, there is also a documented reduction in quality of life with anaemia[23].

A potential issue with all the cohort studies is bias due to unrecognised confounding factors. The cause of anaemia in the general medical population is often multifactorial, and although studies have made allowances for comorbidities, statistical correction may not be adequate, and the haemoglobin may be serving as an indicator of otherwise unaccounted for problems, or their severity.

In chronic kidney disease numerous prospective and retrospective studies have evaluated the effect of haemoglobin concentration on mortality[24-27]. These were reviewed by Volkova and Arab[28], who found a consistent impact of haemoglobin on mortality, although noting heterogeneity between studies and variable degree of control for confounding factors. The relationship between anaemia and mortality remained robust with a haemoglobin level below 110-120g/L, with conclusions unable to be drawn for levels above this. Quality of life is also reduced with anaemia in a number of studies using the SF-36 questionnaire[29].

Cancer patients also have increased risks associated with anaemia. In many malignancies, anaemia is recognised as a prognostic indicator and has been used within prognostic scoring systems, for example in myeloma and Hodgkin disease[30, 31]. Studies across a range of malignancies have shown haemoglobin to be an independent risk factor for reduced survival[32-36]. Anaemia has been shown to impact quality of life in several studies using FACT-An, FACT-F, SF-36 and QLQ-C30 scoring systems[37-39]. Correcting anaemia with erythropoietin stimulating agents has been shown to improve fatigue scores and quality of life in randomised controlled trials[37].

Optimal Haemoglobin Concentration Derived from Population Studies

Population studies may be used to guide optimal haemoglobin levels, where the haemoglobin concentration leading to the best outcomes is considered ideal. In a recent large cohort study Kengne and colleagues found a U-shaped association between cardiovascular and all cause mortality in both diabetic and non-diabetic patients[40]. Interestingly, in patients with diabetes mellitus, anaemia was associated with risk of death similar to that conferred by a prior history of cardiovascular disease. Polycythaemia however conferred a significantly higher risk. The optimal haemoglobin, with the lowest all-cause mortality, was 140g/L. These findings confirm those seen in the Framingham Heart Study, which also showed a U shaped curve with higher mortality and morbidity rates observed at both high and low haematocrit levels[41].

Kunnas and colleagues in the long term follow-up TAMRISK study showed that in males over 50, haematocrits greater than 50% were associated with increased risk of developing cardiovascular disease[42]. The Framingham Heart Study has shown a similar effect, with increasing haematocrit associated with increasing risk of developing cardiac failure, even within the normal range. Indeed in this study, a low haematocrit appeared to protect against the development of cardiac failure[43]. By contrast, in patients with established congestive cardiac failure, anaemia is a consistent risk factor for mortality[18].

The effect of haemoglobin concentration has also been evaluated in pregnant women. Little and colleagues examined a database of women attending for antenatal care within London[44]. There was no correlation with the outcomes and the haemoglobin concentration at the first antenatal check. However the lowest recorded haemoglobin did show a correlation, with a U shaped curve, and the lowest perinatal mortality seen with a haemoglobin concentration between 90-110g/L. This applied both to stillbirths and early neonatal mortality. The reasons for perinatal deaths were not analysed. In pregnancy, despite the low haemoglobin, there is an expanded red cell mass, with a greater increase in plasma volume. The population is also largely a healthy one, without significant cardiorespiratory disease, and therefore ample ability to compensate with increased cardiac output despite relatively low haemoglobin concentrations.

These results demonstrate that across populations anaemia is consistently associated with an increased risk of adverse events and even death. Polycythaemia is associated with a risk of harm. It follows that, at least amongst populations, ideal haemoglobin concentrations to optimise performance or health outcomes may be defined. These may differ between populations. For example haemoglobinopathies associated with a higher oxygen affinity tend to be associated with an increased haematocrit in order to improve oxygen delivery. The case of pregnancy, where an appropriate increase in cardiac output, red cell mass and plasma volume are associated with favourable outcomes, illustrates this point.

Optimising Physical Performance

As the main function of red cells is to carry oxygen, the major symptoms of anaemia, and potential benefit from transfusion relates to oxygen delivery. While haemoglobin concentration is a major factor in determining oxygen delivery to tissues, compensatory mechanisms do exist. Increased cardiac output, alterations in microvascular flow and enhanced oxygen extraction can all potentially buffer oxygen delivery in anaemia. Likewise, an inability to compensate may lead to relatively poor tolerance of anaemia.

The measurement of tissue oxygen delivery is not widely available in the clinic. Measurement of lactate, the product of anaerobic metabolism, can indicate deficient oxygen delivery, but is insensitive to impairment caused by anaemia, being more responsive to tissue hypoperfusion. This may occur as a result of reduced red cell numbers, or decreased total blood volume. Oxygen extraction differs markedly between tissues. The skin and kidneys routinely extract less than 10% of delivered oxygen, whereas the heart extracts 60% of oxygen delivered in healthy non-anaemic individuals. Venous lactate, reflecting large areas of venous drainage from mixed tissues is therefore expected to be a poor indicator of oxygen deficiency within the most sensitive tissues. Based on the relatively high requirement for oxygen, it is expected that the effect of anaemia limiting oxygen delivery will be most noticeable with cardiovascular symptoms.

An "optimal" haemoglobin level, where performance is maximised, has not been defined, but is likely to be much higher than current transfusion guidelines recommend. The optimum haemoglobin level to maximise performance will allow for maximal oxygen delivery, carrying the maximum amount of oxygen within each millilitre of blood, without limiting flow due to increased whole blood viscosity with rising red cell concentration.

Studies in athletes provide evidence of haemoglobin levels that can optimise performance. Recently, Durussel and colleagues examined the effect of recombinant erythropoietin in trained male athletes[45]. Despite having normal haematocrits, the athletes showed a 5-6% improvement in 3000m running time performance when the haematocrit was increased from a mean of 41.9% to 49.2% at the end of a four week course of recombinant erythropoietin. The increased haematocrit and performance was also associated with increased maximal oxygen consumption. Over the subsequent four weeks, performance and measured maximal oxygen consumption decreased with the fall in haematocrit. A similar effect on maximal oxygen consumption has been shown in prior studies[46]. The ergogenic effect appears to be mediated solely by the increase in haemoglobin mass leading to enhanced oxygen carrying capacity, although the widespread presence of erythropoietin receptors within a variety of tissues has fuelled speculation that erythropoietin may have direct ergogenic potential not mediated by increased numbers of red cells.

In a prior study, Brien and Simon demonstrated improved performance over a timed 10km run following autologous transfusion[47]. Each athlete had 2 units (of 450mls each) of whole blood collected at eight week intervals prior to the study, and frozen in glycerol. Washed packed red cells were reinfused in the blinded study, the athletes randomly assigned to packed cells or saline infusions at different times, each occurring 5 days prior to a timed race. Improvements in performance were seen in all athletes following a 400mL packed red cell transfusion, but not with saline. The mean haematocrit after transfusion increased from 41.2% to 47.4%, and performance increased by an average of 69s when the athletes averaged just over 33min at the start of the study.

Although dealing with healthy, well-trained populations, these studies demonstrate a benefit in physiological performance with higher haemoglobin masses within the accepted normal range, and well-above the level usually considered appropriate for transfusion. It is possible that this balance of benefit and risk will vary considerably in disease from that seen in healthy athletes. Increased blood viscosity may impair perfusion in diseased vessels when the haematocrit is higher, and viscosity may be further increased with elevated globulins in chronic inflammatory states.

Assessment of Quality of Life in Anaemia and Transfusion

Symptoms in chronic anaemia have been measured with an anonymous internet based survey of myelodysplastic patients, including validated quality of life assessment, by Steensma and colleagues[48]. They incorporated the FACT-An scale and Brief Fatigue Inventory (BFI) to measure aspects of quality of life. The latter incorporates nine questions measured on a 1-10 scale[49]. Physical capacity was also measured by the Godin Leisure Time Activity Score, which measures the amount of physical activity undertaken over the previous week[50]. Fatigue was the most common symptom reported by patients with myelodysplastic syndrome in this study, but neither the self-reporting of fatigue nor the scores on the BFI or FACT-An scales significantly correlated with anaemia. This appeared to hold true in the population that had never been transfused, suggesting this was not an effect obfuscated by transfusion therapy. Although this type of study has potential for bias and external validation of data, such as the haemoglobin readings reported by patients, could not be undertaken, it is consistent with other data showing poor to moderate correlation between fatigue scores and anaemia, despite this being the most common symptom reported in myelodysplastic syndrome.

Scoring tools have been used to assess anaemia, and in some cases the responses to transfusion. The most common tool used to assess quality of life in the setting of cancer related anaemia is the Functional Assessment of Cancer Therapy – Anaemia (FACT-An) scale. This uses the FACT–G (General) scoring system with additional questions for fatigue (FACT-F subscale) and non-fatigue symptoms of anaemia[51, 52]. It has been used in many studies evaluating the use of erythropoiesis stimulating agents in malignancy and in myelodysplasia. It is well validated in malignancy, with consistency in its association with anaemia noted between studies[53, 54]. It has also been used in myelodysplastic syndrome[55, 56], although its validity has been questioned[57]. Importantly, in cancer and myelodysplasia it shows correlations with the degree of anaemia and responds to haemoglobin increments with erythropoiesis stimulating agents[58]. The European Organisation for Research and Treatment of Cancer (EORTC) QLQ-C30 has been used in a number of studies to evaluate the impact of anaemia, and pharmacological interventions to treat anaemia and myelodysplastic syndromes[38, 56, 59, 60].

In the palliative care setting the Edmonton Symptom Assessment Scale showed a significant improvement in patients transfused with haemoglobin levels less than 80g/L two days after transfusion[61]. Scores for overall wellbeing, fatigue and dyspnoea all improved with transfusion, as did haemoglobin levels. Amongst the group there was only a small, non-significant decline in mean haemoglobin levels by day 15 post transfusion, but a significant fall in quality life, although it remained better than pre-transfusion scores. These results suggest factors other than the haemoglobin concentration may have caused a deterioration in quality of life. Whether this would be seen in chronic anaemia outside of the palliative care setting is not known, as it is possible that declining general health related to the underlying disease may have contributed to falling quality of life scores. The study did not find any differences related to survival time, as might be expected if patients with more advanced disease received less benefit due to comorbidities. It does indicate the potential for comorbidities to confound assessment of symptoms of anaemia using quality of life scores.

The only scoring system specifically devised for myelodysplastic syndrome is QOL-E. It has two general items related to well-being and 26 items addressing functional, physical, fatigue, social and sexual domains[55, 57, 62]. It also has items, such as reference to the perception of regular transfusion on quality of life, that pertain particularly to myelodysplastic syndrome. It does correlate with other quality of life tools, particularly the EQ-5D, a validated and standardised general quality of life score designed to be non-disease specific[63, 64]. It also correlates with anaemia, and independently with transfusion dependence.

The association between quality of life and transfusion dependence itself, independently of anaemia, in this study suggests that transfusion may adversely impact quality of life[57]. Potential causes for this include symptoms associated with transfusions, such as dyspnoea from fluid overload, the need for chelation therapy, the time taken for transfusion, the impact of blood testing or cannulation, or even the impact that having to attend for transfusion has on an individual's perception of their disease. As this study was observational, it may also reflect that the decision to prescribe blood transfusion may be influenced by the degree of quality of life impairment.

The same authors have also compared the quality of life reported by patients with myelodysplastic syndrome with the perceptions of treating clinicians[62]. Clinicians generally rated physical functioning better than patients. Of the patients physicians rated as having Eastern Co-operative Oncology Group (ECOG) functional scores of zero, being fully active with excellent functioning, half rated their own quality of life poorly. This suggests a mismatch between physician assessment and patient perception of their own quality of life. This is an important observation as current guidelines recommend transfusion based on symptoms and in clinical practice these are largely assessed clinically by physicians rather than with a structured tool.

The Short Form 36 (SF 36) is a general quality of life score, with 36 questions covering health eight dimensions[65]. The Multidimensional Fatigue Inventory (MFI) is a 20 question score assessing physical and mental fatigue as well as activity and motivation[66]. Jansen used these two general scores in conjunction with a visual analogue scale (VAS) derived from the European Organisation for the EQ-5D describing "own health today" in myelodysplastic patients[55]. The VAS, physical fatigue and functioning, vitality and reduced functioning domains as measured by the respective scales showed a correlation with anaemia, although in most cases the correlation was weak to moderate. The potential benefit of the visual analogue score for application to clinical practice is its ease of use and simplicity of interpretation. Further studies to validate this approach to assessing quality of life in transfusion are warranted.

Quality of life tools have the advantage of being able to score the symptoms of patients, including physical, emotional and social domains. This is advantageous when there may be quite diverse impacts of diseases and treatments. For example, in the chronically anaemic patient, fatigue and the inconvenience of days in hospital for transfusion may be competing symptoms. This has been borne out in the studies to date, where correlations between scores and haemoglobin levels were present, but weak, suggesting other factors impacting upon the quality of life scores. Each score does have its own weighting for the respective domains, which may or may not reflect a particular patient's priorities. They are also lengthy and cumbersome. In studies where follow up scores were obtained, these were generally infrequent and in many cases had high rates of attrition for the follow up scores. They are therefore generally not applicable to day to day management of patients, and although they would be invaluable for studies in transfusion, as yet they have limited evidence for guiding transfusion in practice.

Quality of life tools have also been used in the acute setting when transfusion is being used to improve functional outcomes. Prick and colleagues have recently demonstrated a small benefit in quality of life from transfusion in women with anaemia due to severe post-partum haemorrhage, as measured by the Multidimensional Fatigue Index[67]. The study was designed as a non-inferiority study, and was negative, in that a small improvement in MFI score was found at day 3 in the group randomised to transfusion. The authors concluded however that the difference was small and in their view, not clinically meaningful. This may especially be the case in post-partum anaemia where a rapid improvement in haemoglobin concentrations is expected, especially with adequate correction of any underlying iron deficiency. Nevertheless, the study shows the potential to measure quality of life outcomes in transfusion, and has demonstrated a real, albeit small, improvement in fatigue scores in young, and we would assume otherwise mostly fit individuals, transfused for moderate anaemia.

A major difficulty in measuring symptoms as a guide to the need for transfusion, either by formal testing or by clinical assessment, is the potential for concurrent conditions to affect symptoms. Meyers and colleagues looked at quality of life and fatigue in patients with acute myeloid leukaemia and myelodysplastic syndrome before therapy and one month later[68]. Using the Brief Fatigue Inventory a correlation between fatigue and interleukin-1, interleukin-6 and tumour necrosis factor alpha was found prior to therapy, but not with anaemia. Prieto and colleagues looked at fatigue during stem cell transplantation. Using energy level as a single-item construct for physical fatigue, they looked for correlation with clinical features[69]. Performance score, loss of appetite, and depression measured on the Hospital Anxiety and Depression Scale (HADS) and current cigarette smoking were all more strongly associated with reduced energy levels than anaemia.

Transfusion to correct symptoms of anaemia has been studied in advanced cancer. Although there are no randomised trials, studies have assessed the effect of transfusion with validated tools in both prospective and retrospective designs[61, 70-72]. Fatigue has been assessed using the Functional Assessment of Cancer Therapy scales for fatigue (FACT-F) and anaemia (FACT-An) and the Edmonton Symptoms Assessment Scale to determine the effect on fatigue. Although there were mixed results, improvement in fatigue scores, breathlessness and quality of life appeared to improve by the day after transfusion, and lasted for up to 14 days. Not all patients responded, and the overall performance status did not improve, perhaps as the populations studied with advanced cancer had comorbidities or other effects of cancer impacting on performance. In these studies patients started with mean haemoglobin readings of 71-84g/L, and most patients received 2 units of blood to increase the haemoglobin level to around 100g/L[72].

In myelodysplastic syndromes, transfusion guidelines suggest that a haemoglobin target of 100g/L or less is appropriate[3-5]. There are however few studies to support a particular target. There are concerns that transfusing to higher levels will increase the amount of blood required to maintain the higher red cell counts. There are concerns that this may adversely impact the blood supply and increase the rate of iron accumulation. However, there has been no comparison between the red cell needs to maintain higher haemoglobin levels in chronically transfused patients. Nilsson-Ehle and colleagues have found when targeting a haemoglobin of 120g/L that after the initial increase in red cells required to elevate the haemoglobin into this range, there appeared to be no increase in the number of units required to maintain this level compared with the pre-intervention level targeting around 90-100g/L[73]. However, this study was not specifically designed to investigate red cell requirements for different haemoglobin targets, so was not powered to detect a difference in red cell requirements. The results are also confounded by the studies primary aim to assess the effect of darbopoietin. The lack of an increased need for red cells should therefore be treated with caution.

Assessment of Performance in Anaemia

As with athletes, other tools that may be used to assess the impact of anaemia include tests of physical capacity. However a 10km run would not be appropriate for most individuals, especially those with chronic disease. Assessments of maximal oxygen consumption by formal exercise testing are cumbersome. To be used in clinical practice a test needs to be simple and easy to use, reliably reproducible and be correlate with the haemoglobin in any individual. The six minute walk test is a simple test where patients walk at their own pace to cover the greatest distance they can within six minutes, under the supervision of a qualified technician offering encouragement. It has been used in a variety of cardiorespiratory settings where it has been found to be highly reproducible. It correlates with prognosis in congestive cardiac failure, chronic obstructive pulmonary disease and pulmonary hypertension. It also correlates with functional state in these conditions as well as in peripheral vascular disease, fibromyalgia and in the elderly[74]. It is not a measure of maximal performance, but as it is self-paced, may be regarded as a better measurement of the ability to carry out activities of daily living, which are also self-paced and usually not carried out maximal capacity.

The six minute walk test has been used to assess the functional capacity of patients post-operatively and does show a correlation with haemoglobin levels. This association only became significant in post-operative cardiac surgical patients when the haemoglobin fell below 100-105g/L[75]. Although exercise performance fell with lower haemoglobin concentrations, even down to 80g/L, performance on the six minute walk test was considered adequate by the authors for patients to actively participate in their rehabilitation programs. Results after orthopaedic surgery have been conflicting, with some studies showing an association and others indicating no association between six minute walking distance and haemoglobin[76]. In congestive cardiac failure, haemoglobin does appear to be associated with the six minute walk distance[77, 78], but whether this is improved by transfusion has not been studied.

Although the six minute walk test offers a potential mechanism to quantify functional impairment from anaemia, and response to transfusion, it has been used in only a limited number of studies to date. It has the disadvantages of requiring a patient to attend for a test in a controlled environment with adequate professional supervision for the duration. Furthermore, the test does not indicate the cause for functional impairment, which may be from a variety of cardiorespiratory, mechanical or other comorbidities.

Performance in treadmill exercise stress testing has, in a manner similar to the six minute walk, been associated with haemoglobin[79]. No studies have evaluated exercise stress testing as a means to measure response to transfusion. Wallis and colleagues have also recently used bicycle ergometric tests to show that transfusion improves exercise performance with a greater capacity to exercise before reaching the anaerobic threshold in haematology patients undergoing chronic transfusion[80]. Such a technique may be useful in future studies to help determine or validate transfusion thresholds, but formal exercise performance testing is an intensive tool for routine clinical practice.

Other Indicators of the Need for Transfusion

Measures of tissue hypoxia, such as lactate, rise late in tissue hypoxia, and are not usually increased with anaemia, being a better measure for hypoperfusion than early hypoxia. Near infra-red spectroscopy is a technique used to measure oxygen delivery to the capillary bed[81]. Using infra-red light, which is absorbed by deoxygenated blood, and near infra-red light, which is absorbed by both oxygenated and deoxygenated blood, the test is able to measure deeper into tissues as it is not absorbed by bone, skin or other organs. It can therefore measure oxygenation within organs such as the brain.

The measurement of arterial oxygen saturation is a widely undertaken and simple procedure with pulse oximeters. As they measure only the proportion of oxy and deoxy- haemoglobin they cannot measure anaemia. The measurement occurs before the tissue vascular bed, so they function as a measure of oxygen transport from the lungs, and do not reflect the oxygen delivery to tissues. Unlike pulse oximetry, near infra-red spectroscopy evaluates oxygenation deeper in tissues, and can therefore assess organ ischaemia. As such it has been assessed in the setting of acute blood loss to determine the effect on tissue oxygenation. Reduced levels may be decreased for a number of reasons, including vascular impairment, hypovolaemia and anaemia. Its emerging role has been recently reviewed by Hampton and Schreiber[81].

Torella and colleagues evaluated near infra-red spectroscopy in the setting of acute normovolaemic haemodilution pre-operatively and found a correlation with the fall in haemoglobin and both gastrocnemius muscle and cerebral cortex measurements of oxygen saturation[82]. These changes occurred with haemodilution only down to a target of 11g/L. In another study, they have demonstrated an improvement in oxygen saturation as measured by near infra-red spectroscopy with transfusion[83]. It has been used to detect hypoperfusion in the setting of cardiac surgery, resuscitation following trauma and in abdominal surgery. One study in neonates has shown no improvement in tissue oxygenation with transfusion, despite improvements in the number of bradycardic events. The transfusion threshold in this study was 80+/- 9g/L.

Although it has not been used in the chronic setting, the ability to observe changes in tissue oxygenation suggests this emerging technique could potentially be applied to patients with long term anaemia to objectively measure changes that may signify the need for transfusion. Evidence from the acute setting, where tissue hypoxia may occur from poor perfusion rather than anaemia, should be interpreted with caution in the chronic transfusion setting. Near infra-red spectroscopy provides an instantaneous assessment of tissue hypoxia and it would be anticipated that results in anaemic patients may vary at rest or with exertion. Nevertheless, it appears to be a promising tool in need of further evaluation.

Conclusion

There are a large number of patients with chronic anaemia from medical causes such myelodysplasia for whom transfusion is considered as therapy.

Despite the use of transfusion therapy for over a century, evidence for the optimal approach to chronic transfusion remains poor. Physicians prescribing blood need to draw on evidence from a variety of sources, and guidelines developed by a variety of groups.

Particular groups, such as thalassaemia and sickle cell disease, have guidelines developed based on avoiding known complications to occur in these groups, which while providing some guidance, may have limited applicability to adults without these conditions. Population based studies indicate increased risk of adverse outcomes associated with lower haemoglobin levels, with the optimal haemoglobin varying with the particular characteristics of populations studied.

It cannot be assumed though that correcting anaemia will lead to improvement in outcomes simply because population studies show anaemia is a risk factor. Recombinant human erythropoietin therapy has been associated with now well-established risks when administered to achieve haemoglobin levels within the normal range. These findings were unexpected, as initial studies were of short term duration and evaluated only quality of life, and caution needs to be exercised to avoid duplicating this in the field of red cell transfusion. Controlled prospective studies are needed to show effectiveness of interventions to correct anaemia, as there are plenty of data pointing to potential harm from transfusion.

The optimal haemoglobin to improve performance has been studied in athletes and is higher than current transfusion guidelines would consider a reasonable level for transfusion therapy. This is not unreasonable as most patients are requiring haemoglobin levels adequate to avoid symptoms of anaemia during activities of daily living rather than aiming to enhance their peak performance potential. Relatively simple tests, such as the validated six minute walk test, have the potential to measure functional improvement or otherwise associated with transfusion. Quality of life tools may be more appropriate to measure the impact of anaemia in medical patients, and have been used widely in the study of erythropoietin, and to a lesser extent in transfusion. These have the advantage of taking into account the physiological limitations encountered with transfusion, but also the patients' needs in undertaking their usual activities, rather than an arbitrary physiological value. There is a need for further research into the most appropriate, simple tools for assessing the impact of anaemia and the benefit of transfusion. This should focus on identifying novel objective transfusion triggers that could be used, perhaps in an individualised way, that take into account the needs of the blood recipient rather than somewhat arbitrary haemoglobin values.

References

[1] Kassebaum, NJ; Jasrasaria, R; Naghavi, M; Wulf, SK; Johns, N; Lozano, R. et al. A systematic analysis of global anemia burden from 1990 to 2010. *Blood*. 2013 December 2, 2013.

[2] Crispin, P. Transfusion Reactions Hidden From History. *Hektoen International*. 2014, Accepted.

[3] Szczepiorkowski, ZM; Dunbar, NM. Transfusion guidelines: when to transfuse. *Hematology Am Soc Hematol Educ Program*. 2013, 2013, 638-44.

[4] National_Blood_Authority. Patient Blood Management Guidelines: Module 3 Medical. Canberra: National Blod Authority, 2012.

[5] Carson, JL; Grossman, BJ; Kleinman, S; Tinmouth, AT; Marques, MB; Fung, MK; et al. Red blood cell transfusion: a clinical practice guideline from the AABB*. *Ann Intern Med*. 2012 Jul 3, 157(1), 49-58.

[6] Qaseem, A; Humphrey, LL; Fitterman, N; Starkey, M; Shekelle, P. Treatment of anemia in patients with heart disease: a clinical practice guideline from the American College of Physicians. *Ann Intern Med*. 2013 Dec 3, 159(11), 770-9.

[7] Villanueva, C; Colomo, A; Bosch, A; Concepcion, M; Hernandez-Gea, V; Aracil, C; et al. Transfusion strategies for acute upper gastrointestinal bleeding. *N Engl J Med*. 2013 Jan 3, 368(1), 11-21.

[8] Hebert, PC; Wells, G; Blajchman, MA; Marshall, J; Martin, C; Pagliarello, G; et al. A multicenter, randomized, controlled clinical trial of transfusion requirements in critical care. Transfusion Requirements in Critical Care Investigators, Canadian Critical Care Trials Group. *N Engl J Med*. 1999 Feb 11, 340(6), 409-17.

[9] Lacroix, J; Hebert, PC; Hutchison, JS; Hume, HA; Tucci, M; Ducruet, T; et al. Transfusion strategies for patients in pediatric intensive care units. *N Engl J Med*. 2007 Apr 19, 356(16), 1609-19.

[10] Josephson, CD; Su, LL; Hillyer, KL; Hillyer, CD. Transfusion in the patient with sickle cell disease: a critical review of the literature and transfusion guidelines. *Transfus Med Rev*. 2007 Apr, 21(2), 118-33.

[11] Musallam, KM; Angastiniotis, M; Eleftheriou, A; Porter, JB. Cross-talk between available guidelines for the management of patients with beta-thalassemia major. *Acta Haematol*. 2013, 130(2), 64-73.

[12] Priddee, NR; Pendry, K; Ryan, KE. Fresh blood for transfusion in adults with beta thalassaemia. *Transfus Med*. 2011 Dec, 21(6), 417-20.

[13] Telfer, P. Update on survival in thalassemia major. *Hemoglobin.* 2009, 33 Suppl 1, S76-80.
[14] Brittenham, GM. Iron-Chelating Therapy for Transfusional Iron Overload. *New England Journal of Medicine.* 2011, 364(2), 146-56.
[15] National_Blood_Authority. Patient Blood Management Guideline: Module 1 – Critical Bleeding/Massive Transfusion. Canberra: National Blood Authority, 2011.
[16] Ennezat, PV; Marechaux, S; Pincon, C; Finzi, J; Barrailler, S; Bouabdallaoui, N; et al. Anaemia to predict outcome in patients with acute coronary syndromes. *Arch Cardiovasc Dis.* 2013 Jun-Jul, 106(6-7), 357-65.
[17] Lawler, PR; Filion, KB; Dourian, T; Atallah, R; Garfinkle, M; Eisenberg, MJ. Anemia and mortality in acute coronary syndromes: a systematic review and meta-analysis. *Am Heart J.* 2013 Feb, 165(2), 143-53 e5.
[18] Barlera, S; Tavazzi, L; Franzosi, MG; Marchioli, R; Raimondi, E; Masson, S. et al. Predictors of mortality in 6975 patients with chronic heart failure in the Gruppo Italiano per lo Studio della Streptochinasi nell'Infarto Miocardico-Heart Failure trial: proposal for a nomogram. *Circ Heart Fail.* 2013 Jan, 6(1), 31-9.
[19] Levy, WC; Mozaffarian, D; Linker, DT; Sutradhar, SC; Anker, SD; Cropp, AB; et al. The Seattle Heart Failure Model: Prediction of Survival in Heart Failure. *Circulation.* 2006 March 21, 2006, 113(11), 1424-33.
[20] Adams, KF; Jr. Pina, IL; Ghali, JK; Wagoner, LE; Dunlap, SH; Schwartz, TA; et al. Prospective evaluation of the association between hemoglobin concentration and quality of life in patients with heart failure. *Am Heart J.* 2009 Dec, 158(6), 965-71.
[21] Anand, IS; Kuskowski, MA; Rector, TS; Florea, VG; Glazer, RD; Hester, A; et al. Anemia and change in hemoglobin over time related to mortality and morbidity in patients with chronic heart failure: results from Val-HeFT. *Circulation.* 2005 Aug 23, 112(8), 1121-7.
[22] Kalra, PR; Collier, T; Cowie, MR; Fox, KF; Wood, DA; Poole-Wilson, PA; et al. Haemoglobin concentration and prognosis in new cases of heart failure. *Lancet.* 2003 Jul 19, 362(9379), 211-2.
[23] Iqbal, J; Francis, L; Reid, J; Murray, S; Denvir, M. Quality of life in patients with chronic heart failure and their carers: a 3-year follow-up study assessing hospitalization and mortality. *Eur J Heart Fail.* 2010 Sep, 12(9), 1002-8.

[24] Astor, BC; Coresh, J; Heiss, G; Pettitt, D; Sarnak, MJ. Kidney function and anemia as risk factors for coronary heart disease and mortality: the Atherosclerosis Risk in Communities (ARIC) Study. *Am Heart J.* 2006 Feb, 151(2), 492-500.
[25] Avram, MM; Blaustein, D; Fein, PA; Goel, N; Chattopadhyay, J; Mittman, N. Hemoglobin predicts long-term survival in dialysis patients: a 15-year single-center longitudinal study and a correlation trend between prealbumin and hemoglobin. *Kidney Int Suppl.* 2003 Nov(87), S6-11.
[26] Abramson, JL; Jurkovitz, CT; Vaccarino, V; Weintraub, WS; McClellan, W. Chronic kidney disease, anemia, and incident stroke in a middle-aged, community-based population: the ARIC Study. *Kidney Int.* 2003 Aug, 64(2), 610-5.
[27] Jurkovitz, CT; Abramson, JL; Vaccarino, LV; Weintraub, WS; McClellan, WM. Association of high serum creatinine and anemia increases the risk of coronary events: results from the prospective community-based atherosclerosis risk in communities (ARIC) study. *J Am Soc Nephrol.* 2003 Nov, 14(11), 2919-25.
[28] Volkova, N; Arab, L. Evidence-based systematic literature review of hemoglobin/hematocrit and all-cause mortality in dialysis patients. *Am J Kidney Dis.* 2006 Jan, 47(1), 24-36.
[29] Finkelstein, FO; Story, K; Firanek, C; Mendelssohn, D; Barre, P; Takano, T; et al. Health-related quality of life and hemoglobin levels in chronic kidney disease patients. *Clin J Am Soc Nephrol.* 2009 Jan, 4(1), 33-8.
[30] Durie, BG; Salmon, SE. A clinical staging system for multiple myeloma. Correlation of measured myeloma cell mass with presenting clinical features, response to treatment, and survival. *Cancer.* 1975 Sep, 36(3), 842-54.
[31] Hasenclever, D; Diehl, V; Armitage, JO; Assouline, D; Björkholm, M; Brusamolino, E et al. A Prognostic Score for Advanced Hodgkin's Disease. *New England Journal of Medicine.* 1998, 339(21), 1506-14.
[32] Caro, JJ; Salas, M; Ward, A; Goss, G. Anemia as an independent prognostic factor for survival in patients with cancer: a systemic, quantitative review. *Cancer.* 2001 Jun 15, 91(12), 2214-21.
[33] Beer, TM; Tangen, CM; Bland, LB; Hussain, M; Goldman, BH; DeLoughery, TG; et al. The prognostic value of hemoglobin change after initiating androgen-deprivation therapy for newly diagnosed

metastatic prostate cancer: A multivariate analysis of Southwest Oncology Group Study 8894. *Cancer.* 2006 Aug 1, 107(3), 489-96.
[34] Mandrekar, SJ; Schild, SE; Hillman, SL; Allen, KL; Marks, RS; Mailliard, JA; et al. A prognostic model for advanced stage nonsmall cell lung cancer. Pooled analysis of North Central Cancer Treatment Group trials. *Cancer.* 2006 Aug 15, 107(4), 781-92.
[35] Kohne, CH; Cunningham, D; Di, Costanzo, F; Glimelius, B; Blijham, G; Aranda, E; et al. Clinical determinants of survival in patients with 5-fluorouracil-based treatment for metastatic colorectal cancer: results of a multivariate analysis of 3825 patients. *Ann Oncol.* 2002 Feb, 13(2), 308-17.
[36] Negrier, S; Escudier, B; Gomez, F; Douillard, JY; Ravaud, A; Chevreau, C; et al. Prognostic factors of survival and rapid progression in 782 patients with metastatic renal carcinomas treated by cytokines: a report from the Groupe Francais d'Immunotherapie. *Ann Oncol.* 2002 Sep, 13(9), 1460-8.
[37] Tonia, T; Mettler, A; Robert, N; Schwarzer, G; Seidenfeld, J; Weingart, O; et al. Erythropoietin or darbepoetin for patients with cancer. *Cochrane Database Syst Rev.* 2012, 12:CD003407.
[38] Wisloff, F; Gulbrandsen, N; Hjorth, M; Lenhoff, S; Fayers, P. Quality of life may be affected more by disease parameters and response to therapy than by haemoglobin changes. *Eur J Haematol.* 2005 Oct, 75(4), 293-8.
[39] Nieboer, P; Buijs, C; Rodenhuis, S; Seynaeve, C; Beex, LV; van, der, Wall, E; et al. Fatigue and relating factors in high-risk breast cancer patients treated with adjuvant standard or high-dose chemotherapy: a longitudinal study. *J Clin Oncol.* 2005 Nov 20, 23(33), 8296-304.
[40] Kengne, AP; Czernichow, S; Hamer, M; Batty, GD; Stamatakis, E. Anaemia, haemoglobin level and cause-specific mortality in people with and without diabetes. *PLoS One.* 2012, 7(8), e41875.
[41] Gagnon, DR; Zhang, TJ; Brand, FN; Kannel, WB. Hematocrit and the risk of cardiovascular disease--the Framingham study: a 34-year follow-up. *Am Heart J.* 1994 Mar, 127(3), 674-82.
[42] Kunnas, T; Solakivi, T; Huuskonen, K; Kalela, A; Renko, J; Nikkari, ST. Hematocrit and the risk of coronary heart disease mortality in the TAMRISK study, a 28-year follow-up. Prev Med. 2009 Aug, 49(1), 45-7.
[43] Coglianese, EE; Qureshi, MM; Vasan, RS; Wang, TJ; Moore, LL. Usefulness of the blood hematocrit level to predict development of heart failure in a community. *Am J Cardiol.* 2012 Jan 15, 109(2), 241-5.

[44] Little, MP; Brocard, P; Elliott, P; Steer, PJ. Hemoglobin concentration in pregnancy and perinatal mortality: a London-based cohort study. *Am J Obstet Gynecol*. 2005 Jul, 193(1), 220-6.

[45] Durussel, J; Daskalaki, E; Anderson, M; Chatterji, T; Wondimu, DH; Padmanabhan, N; et al. Haemoglobin mass and running time trial performance after recombinant human erythropoietin administration in trained men. *PLoS One*. 2013, 8(2), e56151.

[46] Russell, G; Gore, CJ; Ashenden, MJ; Parisotto, R; Hahn, AG. Effects of prolonged low doses of recombinant human erythropoietin during submaximal and maximal exercise. *Eur J Appl Physiol*. 2002 Mar, 86(5), 442-9.

[47] Brien, AJ; Simon, TL. The effects of red blood cell infusion on 10-km race time. *JAMA*. 1987 May 22-29, 257(20), 2761-5.

[48] Steensma, DP; Heptinstall, KV; Johnson, VM; Novotny, PJ; Sloan, JA; Camoriano, JK; et al. Common troublesome symptoms and their impact on quality of life in patients with myelodysplastic syndromes (MDS), results of a large internet-based survey. *Leuk Res*. 2008 May, 32(5), 691-8.

[49] Mendoza, TR; Wang, XS; Cleeland, CS; Morrissey, M; Johnson, BA; Wendt, JK; et al. The rapid assessment of fatigue severity in cancer patients: use of the Brief Fatigue Inventory. *Cancer*. 1999 Mar 1, 85(5), 1186-96.

[50] Godin, G; Shephard, RJ. A simple method to assess exercise behavior in the community. *Can J Appl Sport Sci*. 1985 Sep, 10(3), 141-6.

[51] Yellen, SB; Cella, DF; Webster, K; Blendowski, C; Kaplan, E. Measuring fatigue and other anemia-related symptoms with the Functional Assessment of Cancer Therapy (FACT) measurement system. *Journal of pain and symptom management*. 1997, 13(2), 63-74.

[52] Cella, D; Eton, DT; Lai, J-S; Peterman, AH; Merkel, DE. Combining Anchor and Distribution-Based Methods to Derive Minimal Clinically Important Differences on the Functional Assessment of Cancer Therapy (FACT) Anemia and Fatigue Scales. *Journal of pain and symptom management*. 2002, 24(6), 547-61.

[53] Wasada, I; Eguchi, H; Kurita, M; Kudo, S; Shishida, T; Mishima, Y; et al. Anemia affects the quality of life of Japanese cancer patients. *Tokai J Exp Clin Med*. 2013 Apr, 38(1), 7-11.

[54] Bremberg, ER; Brandberg, Y; Hising, C; Friesland, S; Eksborg, S. Anemia and quality of life including anemia-related symptoms in

patients with solid tumors in clinical practice. *Med Oncol.* 2007, 24(1), 95-102.

[55] Jansen, AJ; Essink-Bot, ML; Beckers, EA; Hop, WC; Schipperus, MR; Van, Rhenen, DJ. Quality of life measurement in patients with transfusion-dependent myelodysplastic syndromes. *Br J Haematol.* 2003 Apr, 121(2), 270-4.

[56] Pinchon, DJ; Stanworth, SJ; Doree, C; Brunskill, S; Norfolk, DR. Quality of life and use of red cell transfusion in patients with myelodysplastic syndromes. A systematic review. *Am J Hematol.* 2009 Oct, 84(10), 671-7.

[57] Oliva, EN; D'Angelo, A; Martino, B; Nobile, F; Dimitrov, BD; Perna, A. More concern about transfusion requirement when evaluating quality of life in anemic patients. *J Clin Oncol.* 2002 Jul 15, 20(14), 3182-3, author reply 3-4.

[58] Spiriti, MA; Latagliata, R; Niscola, P; Cortelezzi, A; Francesconi, M; Ferrari, D; et al. Impact of a new dosing regimen of epoetin alfa on quality of life and anemia in patients with low-risk myelodysplastic syndrome. *Ann Hematol.* 2005 Mar, 84(3), 167-76.

[59] Aaronson, NK; Ahmedzai, S; Bergman, B; Bullinger, M; Cull, A; Duez, NJ; et al. The European Organization for Research and Treatment of Cancer QLQ-C30: a quality-of-life instrument for use in international clinical trials in oncology. *J Natl Cancer Inst.* 1993 Mar 3, 85(5), 365-76.

[60] Kantarjian, H; Issa, J-PJ; Rosenfeld, CS; Bennett, JM; Albitar, M; DiPersio, J; et al. Decitabine improves patient outcomes in myelodysplastic syndromes. *Cancer.* 2006, 106(8), 1794-803.

[61] Mercadante, S; Ferrera, P; Villari, P; David, F; Giarratano, A; Riina, S. Effects of red blood cell transfusion on anemia-related symptoms in patients with cancer. *J Palliat Med.* 2009 Jan, 12(1), 60-3.

[62] Oliva, EN; Finelli, C; Santini, V; Poloni, A; Liso, V; Cilloni, D; et al. Quality of life and physicians' perception in myelodysplastic syndromes. *Am J Blood Res.* 2012, 2(2), 136-47.

[63] Hurst, NP; Kind, P; Ruta, D; Hunter, M; Stubbings, A. Measuring health-related quality of life in rheumatoid arthritis: validity, responsiveness and reliability of EuroQol (EQ-5D). *Br J Rheumatol.* 1997 May, 36(5), 551-9.

[64] Johnson, JA; Coons, SJ; Ergo, A; Szava-Kovats, G. Valuation of EuroQOL (EQ-5D) health states in an adult US sample. *Pharmacoeconomics.* 1998 Apr, 13(4), 421-33.

[65] Ware, JE, Jr., Sherbourne CD. The MOS 36-item short-form health survey (SF-36). I. Conceptual framework and item selection. *Med Care.* 1992 Jun, 30(6), 473-83.
[66] Lin, JM; Brimmer, DJ; Maloney, EM; Nyarko, E; Belue, R; Reeves, WC. Further validation of the Multidimensional Fatigue Inventory in a US adult population sample. *Popul Health Metr.* 2009, 7:18.
[67] Prick, BW; Jansen, AJG; Steegers, EAP; Hop, WCJ; Essink-Bot, ML; Uyl-de, Groot, CA; et al. Transfusion policy after severe postpartum haemorrhage: a randomised non-inferiority trial. *BJOG: An International Journal of Obstetrics & Gynaecology.* 2014:n/a-n/a.
[68] Meyers, CA; Albitar, M; Estey, E. Cognitive impairment, fatigue, and cytokine levels in patients with acute myelogenous leukemia or myelodysplastic syndrome. *Cancer.* 2005, 104(4), 788-93.
[69] Prieto, JM; Blanch, J; Atala, J; Carreras, E; Rovira, M; Cirera, E; et al. Clinical factors associated with fatigue in haematologic cancer patients receiving stem-cell transplantation. *Eur J Cancer.* 2006 Aug, 42(12), 1749-55.
[70] Brown, E; Hurlow, A; Rahman, A; Closs, SJ; Bennett, MI. Assessment of fatigue after blood transfusion in palliative care patients: a feasibility study. *J Palliat Med.* 2010 Nov, 13(11), 1327-30.
[71] Gleeson, C; Spencer, D. Blood transfusion and its benefits in palliative care. *Palliat Med.* 1995 Oct, 9(4), 307-13.
[72] Preston, NJ; Hurlow, A; Brine, J; Bennett, MI. Blood transfusions for anaemia in patients with advanced cancer. *Cochrane Database Syst Rev.* 2012, 2:CD009007.
[73] Nilsson-Ehle, H; Birgegård, G; Samuelsson, J; Antunovic, P; Astermark, J; Garelius, H; et al. Quality of life, physical function and MRI T2* in elderly low-risk MDS patients treated to a haemoglobin level of ≥120 g/L with darbepoetin alfa ± filgrastim or erythrocyte transfusions. *European Journal of Haematology.* 2011, 87(3), 244-52.
[74] ATS statement: guidelines for the six-minute walk test. *Am J Respir Crit Care Med.* 2002 Jul 1, 166(1), 111-7.
[75] Ranucci, M; La, Rovere, MT; Castelvecchio, S; Maestri, R; Menicanti, L; Frigiola, A; et al. Postoperative anemia and exercise tolerance after cardiac operations in patients without transfusion: what hemoglobin level is acceptable? *Ann Thorac Surg.* 2011 Jul, 92(1), 25-31.
[76] Cavenaghi, F; Cerri, C; Panella, L. Association of hemoglobin levels, acute hemoglobin decrease and age with Rehabilitation outcomes after

total hip and knee replacement. *Eur J Phys Rehabil Med.* 2009 Sep, 45(3), 319-25.
[77] Ingle, L; Rigby, AS; Nabb, S; Jones, PK; Clark, AL; Cleland, JG. Clinical determinants of poor six-minute walk test performance in patients with left ventricular systolic dysfunction and no major structural heart disease. *Eur J Heart Fail.* 2006 May, 8(3), 321-5.
[78] Mancini, DM; Katz, SD; Lang, CC; LaManca, J; Hudaihed, A; Androne, AS. Effect of erythropoietin on exercise capacity in patients with moderate to severe chronic heart failure. *Circulation.* 2003 Jan 21, 107(2), 294-9.
[79] Lipinski, MJ; Dewey, FE; Biondi-Zoccai, GG; Abbate, A; Vetrovec, GW; Froelicher, VF. Hemoglobin levels predict exercise performance, ST-segment depression, and outcome in patients referred for routine exercise treadmill testing. *Clin Cardiol.* 2009 Dec, 32(12), E22-31.
[80] Wallis, JP, editor. Physiology of Anaemia and Red Cell Transfusion. Australian and New Zealand Society for Blood Transfusion Annual Scientific Meeting, 2013, Broadbeach.
[81] Hampton, DA; Schreiber, MA. Near infrared spectroscopy: clinical and research uses. *Transfusion.* 2013 Jan, 53 Suppl 1, 52S-8S.
[82] Torella, F; Haynes, SL; McCollum, CN. Cerebral and peripheral near-infrared spectroscopy: an alternative transfusion trigger? *Vox Sang.* 2002 Oct, 83(3), 254-7.
[83] Torella, F; Haynes, SL; McCollum, CN. Cerebral and peripheral oxygen saturation during red cell transfusion. *J Surg Res.* 2003 Mar, 110(1), 217-21.

In: Anemia
Editor: Alice Hallman

ISBN: 978-1-63321-775-1
© 2014 Nova Science Publishers, Inc.

Chapter 7

Anaemia: Prevalence, Risk Factors and Management with a Focus on Chronic Kidney Disease

K. Abdul Razak[1], D.W. Mudge[2] and D. W. Johnson[3]
[1]Department of Nephrology, Princess Alexandra Hospital, Woolloongabba, Queensland, Australia
[2]Department of Nephrology, University of Queensland at Princess Alexandra Hospital, Woolloongabba, Queensland, Australia
[3]Department of Nephrology, University of Queensland at Princess Alexandra Hospital, Woolloongabba, Queensland, Australia

Abstract

The global prevalence of anaemia has decreased over the last 20 years from 40.2% in 1990 to 32.9% in 2010, but with a significant geographical variation. Iron deficiency, the commonest cause, decreased as a proportion, whereas the anaemia of chronic kidney disease increased. Anaemia due to haemoglobinopathies remained relatively constant. The increasing anaemia in kidney disease coupled with ageing and population growth resulted in a dramatic increase in the number of patients in this group. Higher income regions have a higher proportion of haemoglobinopathies, kidney disease and gastrointestinal bleeding. Among the elderly, nutrition, kidney disease and its other associated risk factors (diabetes mellitus, hypertension and cardiovascular disease) were the greatest contributors to anaemia. The focus of this article is iron deficiency anaemia related to kidney disease, its risk factors and management strategies. Iron supplementation remains the cornerstone treatment of iron deficiency and the anaemia of kidney disease. Early and correct diagnosis of iron deficiency along with optimisation of iron stores is also the primary aim of the management of the cardiorenal syndrome and anaemia in diabetes. Recent trials comparing various oral iron formulations have yielded conflicting results. Newer intravenous preparations including ferric carboxymaltose and ferumoxytol have simplified management by permitting safer high-dose administration. Erythropoietin stimulating agents are also established therapy for patients with anaemia and kidney disease, and are used in early kidney disease, diabetes and the cardiorenal syndrome. However recent large trials have raised concern over the safety of these agents in treating anaemia, particularly at high doses.

Introduction

Anaemia is defined as a reduction in one or more of the major red blood cell (RBC) measurements obtained as a part of the complete blood count: haemoglobin (Hb) concentration, haematocrit, or RBC count. Anaemia surveillance is challenging due to marked variation in normal haemoglobin levels with age, gender, ethnicity and socioeconomic background [1]. Its prevalence is also influenced by body weight and physiological state like pregnancy. Anaemia is pathophysiologically diverse and often multifactorial. The World Health Organization (WHO) defines anaemia as a Hb level below 130 g/L in men, 120 g/L in women, and 110 g/L in pregnant women and preschool children. Iron deficiency anaemia (IDA) is the most common form of anaemia worldwide [2]. It is associated with impaired cognitive development in preschool-aged children and diminished work productivity and cognitive and behavioural problems in adults [3, 4]. Among pregnant women, IDA has been associated with increased risks of low birth weight, prematurity and maternal morbidity [5]. IDA is the consequence of iron loss or requirement that exceeds iron supply and absorption. Increase requirement is the result of increased physiological need associated with normal development and hence this category is designated as physiological or nutritional anaemia. Pathological iron deficiency is most often the result of abnormal blood loss or malabsorption. The prevalence of IDA decreased between 1990 and 2010 whereas anaemia of chronic kidney disease (CKD) increased in prevalence. Anaemia from CKD increased with age in an accelerating fashion for both sexes, culminating as the most prevalent cause of anaemia in the 80+ years age group[6]. In developed countries like the United States, the Third National Health and Nutritional Evaluation Survey (NHANES III, 1999-2006) has shown a CKD prevalence of 11.3 % in adult population [7]. The number is increasing with the ageing population and contributory diseases such as diabetes and hypertension becoming more common [8]. This article focuses on pathological causes of IDA with special attention to anaemia in CKD and associated risk factors which are a growing global burden of non-communicable diseases.

Anaemia Prevalence

The global anaemia burden was accounted by Kassebaum et al[6] using data, methods and analytical resources of the Global Burden of Diseases, Injuries and Risk Factors (GBD) Study in 2010.

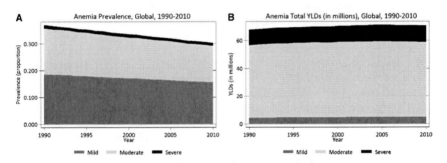

Figure 1. Global anaemia prevalence and total years of life lived with disability (YLD), from 1990 to 2010. Global anaemia burden was calculated for each year from 1980 through 2010 (1980-1990 not shown). Prevalence rates decreased from 40.2% to 32.9% from 1990 to 2010. Roughly two thirds of this decrease can be attributed to decreased sex and cause-specific rates of diseases that lead to anaemia. The remaining one third of the decrease was associated with population aging. Total anaemia burden, as measured in YLD increased from 65.5 to 68.3 million YLD (8.8% of global total from all conditions) from 1990 to 2010. *Republished with permission from[6] Journal of American Society of Hematology; permission conveyed through Copyright Clearance Center, Inc.*

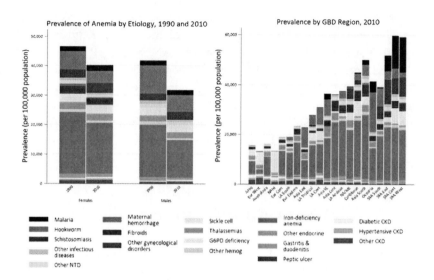

Figure 2: Global and regional cause-specific anaemia prevalence for 1990 and 2010. Prevalence of anaemia for both males and females decreased from 1990 to 2010. The largest improvements for males were in anaemia resulting from hookworm and iron deficiency, while the largest percentage gains for females were in iron deficiency and maternal haemorrhage. Regional differences in proportion of cases resulting from specific causes varied widely. Malaria was a major cause of anaemia in many regions, but none more so than West sub-Saharan Africa, where it accounted for 24.7% of all prevalent anaemia. South and East Asia, despite being among those regions with the greatest reductions in anaemia, had more than half the world's anaemia cases. Anaemia prevalence in 2010 generally increased with decreasing regional mean age of death. Prevalence was highest in East, Central, and West sub-Saharan Africa. These regions also saw the least improvement among all low- and middle-income regions between 1990 and 2010. AP, Asia Pacific; Cent, central; Eur, Europe; G6PD, glucose-6-phosphate dehydrogenase; hemog, hemoglobinemia; HI, high income; LA, Latin America; NA, North America; NA/ME, North Africa/Middle East; NTD, neglected tropical diseases; South, Southern; SE, Southeast; SSA, sub-Saharan Africa.
Republished with permission from[6] Journal of American Society of Hematology; permission conveyed through Copyright Clearance Center, Inc.

Anaemia prevalence has decreased from 40.2% (95% UI, 35.8% to 46.0%) in 1990 to 32.9% (95% UI, 28.9% to 38.5%) in 2010(Figure 1).

There was significant variation in the geographic distribution of anaemia (Figure 2). Higher income regions had the lowest prevalence estimates with major contributions from haemoglobinopathies, CKDs and gastrointestinal haemorrhage.

The causes with highest prevalence in both sexes and all time periods were the same: IDA, parasitic intestinal infections (predominately hookworm), sickle cell disorders, thalassemia, schistosomiasis, and malaria. Global prevalence decreased for most causes between 1990 and 2010. Malaria, schistosomiasis, and CKD were the only causes of anaemia that increased in prevalence, while anaemia as a result of all hemoglobinopathies was relatively static.

Iron Deficiency Anaemia

Iron deficiency was the top ranking cause of anaemia globally (3). Blood loss is the most important cause of iron deficiency in adults. Gastrointestinal (GI) blood loss is the most important cause in men and postmenopausal women and hence a complete endoscopic work up is mandatory. Coeliac disease, *Helicobacter pylori* infection and autoimmune atrophic gastritis have been implicated for refractory IDA. All patients with unexplained refractory IDA should be tested for coeliac disease, *H. pylori* IgG antibodies or faecal antigen, serum gastrin, and antiparietal and intrinsic factor antibodies [9].

Patients with suspected iron deficiency should have iron studies performed and the results correlated with red cell indices.

Table 1 provides guidance for interpretation of results of laboratory tests of iron status.

The serum ferritin level is the most readily available and useful index of iron deficiency. The WHO threshold for diagnosis of iron deficiency in adults is ferritin <15ng/mL, and <12ng/mL for children under five (<30ng/mL where inflammation is coexistent). However, ferritin is also an acute-phase protein and is elevated in inflammation, infection, liver disease and malignancy. Ferritin levels can be misleading in iron-deficient patients with coexisting systemic illness. In the elderly or among patients with inflammation, iron deficiency may still be present with ferritin values up to 60–100 g/L. Measurement of Inflammatory markers such as C-reactive protein (CRP) may help identify coexisting inflammation. Serum iron levels vary significantly with dietary iron intake, circadian rhythm, infection and inflammation. Hence serum iron measurement in isolation should not be used to diagnose iron deficiency [10].

Table 1. Interpreting laboratory blood

Diagnosis	Haemoglobin	Mean cell volume and mean cell haemoglobin	Serum ferritin µg/L	Transferrin or total iron binding capacity	Transferrin saturation†	Soluble transferrin receptor	Serum iron‡
Tissue iron deficiency without anaemia	Normal	Normal or low	< 15–30	Normal or high	Low-normal or low	High-normal or high	Low
Iron deficiency anaemia (IDA)	Low	Low (or normal in early IDA)	< 15–30 adult < 10–12 child	High	Low	High	Low
Anaemia of chronic disease or inflammation	Low	Normal (may be mildly low)	Normal or elevated (elevated ferritin does not imply elevated iron stores)	Normal	Low	Normal	Low
IDA with coexistent chronic disease or inflammation	Low	Low	Low or normal, but usually < 60–100 µg/L	Normal or high	Low	High	Low
Thalassaemia minor§	Low (or normal)	Low (or normal)	Normal or elevated	Normal	Normal or elevated	Normal or elevated	Normal
Iron overload	Normal	Normal	Elevated (correlates with body iron stores)	Normal to low	High	Normal	Normal to elevated

* Compared with laboratory reference range for age, sex and gestation if applicable. † Ideally performed on fasting morning sample. ‡ Serum iron is markedly labile with a significant diurnal variation, is low in both iron deficiency and inflammation, and should not be used to diagnose iron deficiency. § Includes β-thalassaemia minor and single or two alpha gene deletion thalassaemia minor. A thalassaemic condition and iron deficiency may coexist, particularly in pregnancy. Pasricha SRS, Flecknoe-Brown SC et al. Diagnosis and management of iron deficiency anaemia: a clinical update. Med J Aust 2010;193(9):525-532. © Copyright 2010 The Medical Journal of Australia - reproduced with permission.

Functional iron deficiency (FID) is a state in which there is insufficient iron incorporation into erythroid precursors in the face of apparently adequate body iron stores. It is measured by the presence of stainable iron in the bone marrow together with a serum ferritin value within normal limits. FID is commonly seen in CKD patients and is responsible for the suboptimal response to erythropoiesis stimulating agents (ESAs). FID and the partial block in iron transport to the erythroid marrow seen in subjects with infectious, inflammatory and malignant diseases is a major component of the anaemia of chronic disease [11]. Assessment of FID needs evaluation of variables such as percentage of hypochromic red cells (%HRC), reticulocyte haemoglobin content (CHr), soluble transferrin receptor (sTfR) assay and red cell zinc protoporphyrin concentration [11].

Iron Deficiency Anaemia in Chronic Kidney Disease

Anaemia is a frequent complication of CKD. In addition to erythropoietin deficiency, IDA is an important cause of anaemia in CKD patients. CKD patients can have absolute or functional iron deficiency. Absolute iron deficiency in haemodialysis results primarily from excessive blood loss due to dialysis filter and line blood retention, frequent blood testing, dialysis access bleeding, and surgical blood loss. Shortened erythrocyte survival and the erythropoiesis inhibitory effects of accumulating uremic toxins also contribute to the anaemia of CKD[12]. CKD patients often have chronic inflammation which is associated with increased hepcidin levels, which leads to impaired absorption of iron from the gastrointestinal tract and impaired release of iron from body stores [13], leading to functional iron deficiency as well.

Hepcidin is a small peptide hormone of 25 amino acids, produced and secreted predominantly by hepatocytes, circulates in the bloodstream, and is excreted by the kidneys. Hepcidin is the central mediator of systemic iron homeostasis. Hepcidin regulates systemic iron balance by binding and inducing internalization and degradation of ferroportin, an iron channel on the surface of enterocytes, macrophages, and hepatocytes, which is important in iron export into the plasma [13]. Hepcidin levels are elevated in chronic kidney disease and end-stage kidney disease (ESKD) patients, and reflect the balance of stimulatory factors: reduced renal clearance (glomerular filtration rate [GFR]), inflammation, and iron administration; and inhibitory factors: anaemia, erythropoiesis-stimulating agent (ESA) administration, clearance by dialysis, and hypoxia(Figure 3).

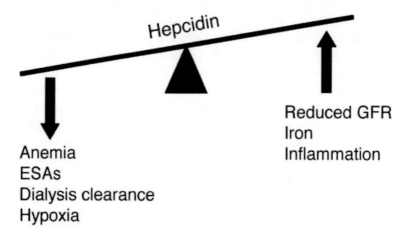

Figure 3. Hepcidin levels in chronic kidney disease and end-stage renal disease patients Hepcidin levels are elevated in chronic kidney disease and end-stage renal disease patients, and reflect the balance of stimulatory factors: reduced renal clearance (GFR, glomerular filtration rate), inflammation, and iron administration; and inhibitory factors: anaemia, erythropoiesis stimulating agent (ESA) administration, clearance by dialysis, and hypoxia. *Reprinted with permission from [13] American Journal of kidney disease.*

Elevated serum hepcidin levels mediate iron-restricted erythropoiesis and contribute to induce anaemia and ESA hyporesponsiveness in CKD patients (10). In CKD, FID can be present when the serum ferritin level is ≥100 ng/ml and a reduction in iron saturation, whereas an absolute IDA is defined a serum ferritin level <100 ng/ml or a transferrin saturation of <20%. The utility of hepcidin measurement as a diagnostic tool is currently uncertain and for the time being this technique remains a research investigation [11].

Anaemia in Diabetes Mellitus

Diabetes is the commonest cause of CKD and therefore renal anaemia. CKD and Type 2 diabetes mellitus frequently coexist, and each disease independently increases the risk of cardiovascular events and end-stage renal disease. Anaemia in diabetes mellitus, particularly in those with CKD, is an independent risk factor for a higher rate of cardiovascular and renal events [14-16]. The data comparison between a 5-year prospective observational study conducted in a diabetes clinic in Australia and the NHANES III survey, found that the prevalence of anaemia in patients with diabetes was 2 to 3 times higher than for patients without diabetes with comparable renal impairment and iron stores. Anaemia in patients with diabetes and CKD worsens with more advanced stages of CKD and in those with proteinuria [15].

Anaemia and the Cardiorenal Syndrome

The cardiorenal syndrome (CRS) is a pathophysiological condition in which combined cardiac and renal dysfunction amplifies progression of failure of the individual organ. At a consensus conference of the Acute Dialysis Quality Initiative (ADQI) in 2010, the CRS was sub-classified into 5 types primarily based upon the organ that initiated the insult as well as the acuity and chronicity of disease [17]. Anaemia is an additional mediator in the progression of either CKD and/or CVD and it is also an independent risk factor for the onset of cardiovascular complications. Anaemia in CRS is multifactorial and is secondary to iron deficiency, chronic inflammation (ACD), dilutional due to salt and water retention, erythropoietin deficiency/resistance and treatment with angiotensin-converting enzyme (ACE) inhibitors or angiotensin-II receptor blockers (ARB). Once considered a complication of heart failure, anaemia is now emerging as a crucial and potentially modifiable factor in the overall treatment strategy for patients with chronic heart failure [18, 19]. Interestingly, one study has shown an improvement in heart failure symptoms in patients treated with parenteral iron, whether or not there was anaemia [20], suggesting iron may have other roles in such patients.

Anaemia in the Elderly

While anaemia prevalence for females decreases steadily with age, anaemia prevalence increases in older males[6](Figure 4). In the third National Health and Nutrition Examination Survey (NHANES III), a nationally representative study [21] of adults aged ≥65 years it was 11.0% in men and 10.2% in women[22]. The prevalence of anaemia in the elderly is drastically greater in the nursing home setting than that in the community setting[23]. Anaemia in the elderly is frequently associated with negative outcomes such as decreased physical performance, increased likelihood of falls, increased frailty, increased hospitalization, increased cognitive impairment and even increased mortality. Pang et al. compared the causes of anaemia in elderly patients in 3 different studies in the US (Figure 5).

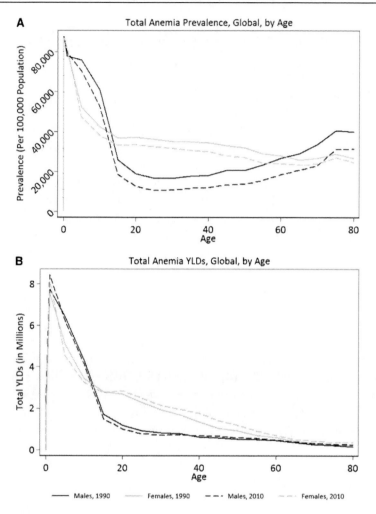

Figure 4. Global burden of anaemia by age. Anaemia burden by age for (A) prevalence and (B) total YLD. Those younger than age 5 years had the highest prevalence and total YLD from anaemia. These age groups also had the least favourable changes between 1990 and 2010. Females had higher prevalence and total YLD than males at all ages. While anaemia prevalence for females decreased steadily with age, anaemia prevalence increased in older age groups among males. As demonstrated by steady decreases in total YLD, however, those prevalent cases among males tended to be less severe. Improvements in anemia prevalence and total YLD for males between 1990 and 2010 were more substantial than those for females although not statistically significant. *Republished with permission from [6] Journal of American Society of Hematology; permission conveyed through Copyright Clearance Center, Inc.*

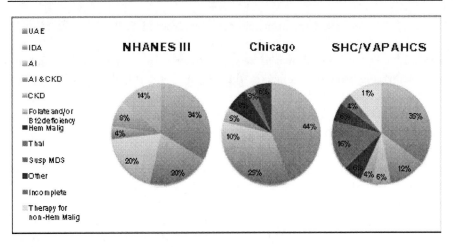

Figure 5. Prevalence of anaemia in the elderly by cause identified in three studies. Studies shown are NHANES III, Chicago and SHC/VAPAHCS. AI, anaemia of inflammation; CKD, anaemia secondary to renal disease; Hem Malig, hematologic malignancy; IDA, iron deficiency anaemia; Susp MDS, suspicious for myelodysplastic syndrome; Thal, thalassemia; UAE, unexplained anaemia of the elderly. *Adapted with permission from Lippincott Williams and Wilkins/Wolters Kluwer Health: Current opinion in Hematology[24].*

The study group differed in their settings where NAHNES III overviewed the prevalence in community dwelling elderly people [24], Artz and Thirman evaluated racially diverse elderly anaemic patients, the majority of whom were African-American women, and Price et al. evaluated elderly anaemic patients who were predominantly white men referred to the Veterans Affairs clinic or referred to a university haematology clinic[21, 24]. The proportion of patients with unexplained anaemia of the elderly (UAE) was similar in these studies. NHANES III did not include other possible underlying causes of anaemia in the elderly, such as myelodysplasia, leukaemia and haemolysis which are important causes in this group. The prevalence of nutrient deficiencies, anaemia of inflammation, and anaemia secondary to renal disease are reduced in the two later studies compared to the NHANES III study.

IDA in the elderly in the Western world is more often due to bleeding and the evaluation of such requires looking beyond poor iron intake, absorption, or processing. The likely source of blood loss in the elderly is the GI tract and a likely source is digestive tract malignancy [25]. The diagnoses of anaemia of inflammation and anaemia secondary to mild renal impairment are very difficult to make, such as when creatinine clearance is 30–60 ml/min. The accurate diagnosis of anaemia of inflammation in the elderly should not rest on arbitrary measurement of iron indices, but should rest on solid clinical findings[24]. Although the serum soluble transferrin receptor (sTfR)–log ferritin index has been shown to be more sensitive than standard iron indices for identifying iron deficiency in the anaemic elderly[21, 26], the regular implementation of this assay is hindered by the lack of standardized reagents for the sTfR assay[27]. The gold standard for diagnosing iron-deficiency anaemia, the absence of iron on an appropriately and adequately stained bone marrow aspirate sample is an invasive method rarely conducted for the sole purpose of differentiating iron deficiency from ACD. Unexplained anaemia of the elderly (UAE) is an entity characterized by a hypoproliferative normocytic anaemia that is not due to the nutritional deficiency, CKD or inflammatory disease; and in which the erythropoietin response to anaemia appears to be blunted. The diagnosis of UAE is usually considered when other causes of anaemia in the elderly have been eliminated [28].

Anaemia Management

Oral Iron Therapy

The WHO recommends that the daily dose of supplemental oral iron should be 60 mg per day to reduce side effects and maximise compliance. The WHO also recommends that the use of ferrous (Fe 2^+) salts is preferable to ferric (Fe 3^+) salt supplements because of greater efficacy and tolerability. Ferrous supplements are also the most cost effective treatment[29]. The major form of oral iron supplement currently used worldwide is ferrous sulphate. Oral iron supplements are associated with the side effects of erosive mucosal injury of the upper gastrointestinal tract as well as nausea, vomiting and epigastric discomfort[30]. Other gastrointestinal side effects include diarrhoea and constipation. These side effects adversely affect treatment compliance and lead to patient withdrawal from treatment[31]. Cancelo-Hidalgo et al. conducted a systematic review to analyse the tolerability of different oral iron supplements [29]. All published data up to January 2009 were analysed. Adverse effects, safety and tolerability of ferrous sulphate, ferrous sulphate with mucoprotease, iron protein succinylate, ferrous fumarate, ferrous gluconate and ferrous glycine sulphate were compared. Extended-release ferrous sulfate with mucoproteose appears to be the best tolerated of the different oral iron supplements evaluated.

Iron (III) Hydroxide Polymaltose Complex

The iron (III)-polymaltose complex is made of non-ionic iron (III), in a form of polynuclear iron (III) hydroxide, and polymaltose ligands. The resulting complex is stable. Being in a non-ionic form, iron does not interact with food components and iron absorption from iron (III) hydroxide polymaltose complex (IPC) appears to be enhanced in the presence of food. Compared to ferrous salts IPC has lower incidence of gastrointestinal side effects [32]. Randomised control trials comparing oral IPC with ferrous salts in pregnant women [33]and paediatric populations [34] has shown oral IPC to be of equivalent efficacy and superior in safety profile compared to ferrous sulphate for the treatment of iron-deficiency. IPC could be a potential focus of research in the field of oral iron therapy in milder or early stages CKD patients.

Newer Oral Iron Therapies

Heme Iron Polypeptide

Heme iron polypeptide (HIP) is a new generation oral iron which uses the haemeporphyrin ring to supply iron to sites of absorption in the intestinal lumen [35]. Heme iron is absorbed via a different receptor to that utilized by non-heme (ionic) iron[36]. Heme iron absorption is not affected by food and high hepcidin levels[37], which potentially makes it an appealing treatment for CKD patients. Nagaraju et al. performed a randomized control trial to compare the efficacy of HIP with IV iron sucrose in the treatment of iron-deficiency anaemia in non-dialysis CKD (ND-CKD) patients. HIP and IV iron sucrose were similar in efficacy in maintaining haemoglobin in ND-CKD patients with no differences in adverse events over 6 months[38]. The HEMATOCRIT trial, a multi-centre, randomized controlled trial of oral heme iron polypeptide versus oral iron supplementation for the treatment of anaemia in peritoneal dialysis population reports differently. In that study, HIP showed no clear safety or efficacy benefit in peritoneal dialysis (PD) patients compared with conventional oral iron supplements. The authors of this study concluded that the reduction in serum ferritin levels and high costs associated with HIP therapy suggest that this agent is unlikely to have a significant role in iron supplementation in PD patients [39].

Erythropoiesis Stimulating Agents

The approval of recombinant human erythropoietin in 1990 facilitated sustained correction of anaemia in CKD. The use of ESAs in CKD patients resulted in progressive rise in haemoglobin concentration from a mean of ~9.5 g/dL to a mean of ~11.5 g/dL, fall in blood transfusions requirement in dialysis units by~50% between 1990 and 2000 (as exemplified by data from the US Renal Data System Report 2009) and dramatic reduction in transfusional iron overload [40](Figure 6).

The currently available erythropoiesis-stimulating agents (ESAs) are epoetin alfa, epoetin beta, darbepoetin alfa, and continuous erythropoietin receptor activator (CERA). Darbepoetin alfa and continuous erythropoietin receptor activator have much longer half-lives and they can be administered less frequently. Peginesatide, a peptide based ESA was approved in the United States in March 2012 for the treatment of anaemia in CKD patients[41] and initially looked promising. However it was withdrawn from the market in 2013 due to reports of fatal hypersensitivity reactions.

The favourable effects of ESA led the wider use of ESAs to earlier stages of chronic kidney disease and anaemia associated with other conditions like diabetes mellitus and cardiorenal anaemia syndrome. ESAs have subsequently been approved in patients undergoing elective surgery and in oncology patients with chemotherapy-induced anaemia[28]. Data from the Correction of Hemoglobin and Outcomes in Renal Insufficiency (CHOIR) trial in which patients received epoetin[42], showed an increase in a composite end point of death and cardiovascular events in the study group receiving a dose targeted to achieve higher haemoglobin levels (13.5 g per decilitre vs. 1.3 g per decilitre). The Trial to Reduce Cardiovascular Events with Aranesp Therapy (TREAT), a randomized, placebo-controlled trial evaluating the cardiovascular benefit with darbepoetin, showed that the risk of stroke increased by a factor of 2 when the targeted haemoglobin level was approximately 13 g per decilitre [43]. Subsequent warnings about ESA prescriptions have led to the revision of anaemia guidelines in CKD. Dialysis Outcomes and Practice Patterns Study (DOPPS) data presented by Bruce Robinson at the National Kidney Foundation Meeting in May 2012 observed that the median haemoglobin levels fell 0.08 g/dL between August 2010 and July 2011, and by an additional 0.37 g/dL up until October 2011. The median weekly ESA dose fell by 28% between August 2010 and December 2011. Intravenous iron use steeply increased from 57% of patients receiving iron in 2010 to 77% in December 2011. More worryingly, the rate of blood transfusions more than doubled from

2.21% of patients transfused per month in September 2010 to 4.87% of patients transfused per month in September 2011 [40].

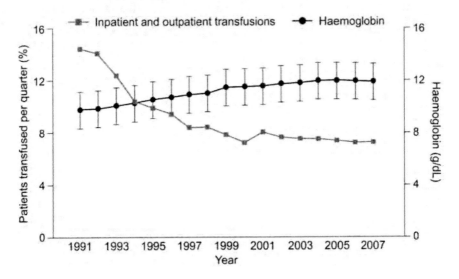

Figure 6. Association of the haemoglobin level and the rate of blood transfusions in US haemodialysis patients 1991–2007. [Data adapted from the US Renal Data System 2009 Annual Report]. *Reproduced by permission of Oxford University Press from [40]Nephrology, dialysis, transplantation.*

Intravenous Iron Treatment

Intravenous (IV) iron treatment has consistently demonstrated to improve the erythropoietic response to ESA treatment. In the dialysis dependant CKD population, the established IV access and convenience of being able to administer IV iron during dialysis treatments are important factors that make IV iron an appropriate choice for iron supplementation[44]. Even in patients with adequate bone marrow iron stores, it is possible to obtain an increase in Hb levels following iron therapy. However, this quantitative effect is lower in patients who are not iron deficient. Stancu et al. showed that, following the administration of 1000 mg of IV iron to 100 patients with ND-CKD, an erythropoietic response was obtained in 63% of those who had iron-deplete bone marrow but only in 30% in those who were iron-replete. The chances of positive response are increased by 7% for each 1% decrease in TSAT [45, 46].

IV iron products currently available for the treatment of iron deficiency in CKD are iron dextran, sodium ferric gluconate, iron sucrose, iron isomaltoside, ferumoxytol and ferric carboxymaltose. The use of IV iron dextran has fallen out of favour in recent years due to the necessity of a test dose and the risk of anaphylactoid reactions even after a successful test dose[47]. Ferumoxytol and ferric carboxymaltose have simplified the management of IDA by permitting faster and higher dose administration without the need for test dose.

Ferumoxytol and Ferric Carboxymaltose

Ferumoxytol is a colloidal iron oxide, coated with a semisynthetic carbohydrate, specifically designed to minimize immunological reactivity. Ferumoxytol has been formulated to be isotonic, eliminating the disadvantages of high osmolality and the need for a prolonged, diluted infusion. Large randomised control trials have proven the efficacy and safety of ferumoxytol in patients with IDA of any underlying cause in whom oral iron cannot be used [48]. It is given as two 510-mg injections 3–8 days apart for a maximum treatment dose of 1020 mg. Ferric carboxymaltose (FCM) is a non-dextran IV iron preparation whose properties permit administration of larger single doses (750 mg) over short periods of time for a maximum treatment dose of 1500 mg [49]. FCM is also proven to be safe and effective in several large trials [50, 51].

Current Treatment Guidelines for Chronic Kidney Disease

The Kidney Disease Improving Global Outcome (KDIGO) Clinical Practice Guideline for Anaemia in Chronic Kidney Disease [52], 2012 recommends:

- When prescribing iron therapy, balance the potential benefits of avoiding or minimizing blood transfusions, ESA therapy, and anaemia-related symptoms against the risks of harm in individual patients (e.g., anaphylactoid and other acute reactions, unknown long-term risks).
- For adult CKD patients with anaemia not on iron or ESA therapy we suggest a trial of IV iron (or in CKD ND patients alternatively a 1–3 month trial of oral iron therapy) if an increase in Hb concentration without starting ESA treatment is desired and TSAT is <30% and ferritin is <500 ng/ml (<500mg/l)

Excessive use of IV iron can theoretically exacerbate oxidative stress, inflammation, endothelial dysfunction, cardiovascular disease, and immune deficiency and potentially increase the risk of microbial infections in this population. Most of these adverse effects are mediated by iron-catalysed generation of reactive oxygen species and the resultant cell injury and dysfunction[53].

Novel Agents for Future Treatment of Anaemia in CKD

Recent safety concerns and limitations of the ESAs have driven research into alternative approaches to mobilize the erythropoietic system. *Roxadustat (FG-4592)* is an orally administered small-molecule inhibitor of hypoxia-inducible factor prolyl hydroxylase (HIF-PH) currently undergoing Phase III trials for the treatment of anaemia in patients with CKD. Hypoxia-inducible factor (HIF) is an oxygen-sensitive transcription factor that mediates cell survival during hypoxic conditions by activating (among other factors) EPO and regulates iron mobilization and utilization[54]. HIF activity is negatively regulated by HIF-PH, so by inhibiting this enzyme FG-4592 prevents the degradation of HIF and stimulates erythropoiesis.

Roxadustat has been shown in clinical studies to correct anaemia and maintain haemoglobin levels without the need for supplementation with intravenous iron in ND-CKD and CKD-5D patients. The data from these ongoing trials are not yet published.

Treatment of Anaemia in Heart Failure and the Elderly

The potential benefits of treating anaemia in patients with heart failure include improved oxygen delivery, attenuation of adverse cardiac remodelling, improved exercise tolerance, and improved health-related quality of life, along with a potential for reduced ischemic myocardial damage by inhibition of myocardial apoptosis.

The Reduction of Events by Darbepoetin Alfa in Heart Failure (RED-HF) trial, randomized, double-blind trial, assigned 2278 patients with systolic heart failure and mild-to-moderate anaemia (haemoglobin level, 9.0 to 12.0 g per decilitre) to receive either darbepoetin alpha (to achieve a haemoglobin target of 13 g per decilitre)or placebo. Treatment with darbepoetin alpha did not improve clinical outcomes in patients with systolic heart failure and mild-to-moderate anaemia [55]. Given the significant risk related to volume overload, blood transfusion is not a first-line therapy, except in patients with severe symptomatic anaemia (haemoglobin<7 g/dL). With the recent evidence linking ESA therapy to achieve high target levels of haemoglobin in anaemic patients with CKD to higher mortality and cardiovascular complications, it would be extremely important to be cautious in utilizing ESAs when treating anaemic patients with heart failure, including the elderly [19].

Conclusion

- Global prevalence of anaemia decreased for most of the causes between 1990 and 2010, whereas anaemia of CKD increased in prevalence. This is the result of increase in ageing population coupled with growing global burden of non-communicable disease like diabetes mellitus and hypertension that contributes to CKD.
- Iron deficiency anaemia, the commonest cause of anaemia world-wide is mostly from GI blood loss in adult men and post-menopausal women warranting a complete GI work up in this population
- Anaemia in CKD is multifactorial. The CKD population has functional iron deficiency mediated by hepcidin and frequently requires the use of erythropoiesis-stimulating agents.
- Anaemia is common in diabetes mellitus with CKD and it increases the risk of cardiorenal syndrome.
- Anaemia prevalence in elderly is higher in men than women. Unexplained anaemia of elderly is the commonest cause of anaemia in elderly population and its evaluation is considerably complex.
- Oral iron therapy is poorly tolerated due to gastrointestinal side effects. Use of newer oral iron preparations are limited by lack of adequate prospective trial evidence, high cost and conflicting results from available literature.
- Safety concerns surrounding ESAs has led to the increased use of IV Iron there by decreasing the ESA requirements.
- The novel oral HIF prolyl hydroxylase inhibitors hold promise for anaemia management in the CKD population.

References

[1] Beutler E, Waalen J: The definition of anemia: what is the lower limit of normal of the blood hemoglobin concentration? *Blood,* 2006, 107(5): 1747- 1750.

[2] McLean E, Cogswell M, Egli I, Wojdyla D, de Benoist B: Worldwide prevalence of anaemia, WHO Vitamin and Mineral Nutrition Information System, 1993-2005. *Public health nutrition,* 2009, 12(4): 444-454.

[3] Sachdev H, Gera T, Nestel P: Effect of iron supplementation on mental and motor development in children: systematic review of randomised controlled trials. *Public health nutrition,* 2005, 8(2):117-132.

[4] Murray-Kolb LE, Beard JL: Iron treatment normalizes cognitive functioning in young women. *The American journal of clinical nutrition,* 2007, 85(3):778-787.

[5] Allen LH: Anemia and iron deficiency: effects on pregnancy outcome. *The American journal of clinical nutrition,* 2000, 71(5 Suppl):1280s-1284s.

[6] Kassebaum NJ, Jasrasaria R, Naghavi M, Wulf SK, Johns N, Lozano R, Regan M, Weatherall D, Chou DP, Eisele TP et al. A systematic analysis of global anemia burden from 1990 to 2010. *Blood,* 2014, 123(5):615-624.

[7] Levey AS, Stevens LA: Estimating GFR using the CKD Epidemiology Collaboration (CKD-EPI) creatinine equation: more accurate GFR estimates, lower CKD prevalence estimates, and better risk predictions. *American journal of kidney diseases : the official journal of the National Kidney Foundation,* 2010, 55(4):622-627.

[8] Coresh J, Selvin E, Stevens LA, Manzi J, Kusek JW, Eggers P, Van Lente F, Levey AS: Prevalence of chronic kidney disease in the United States. *JAMA : the journal of the American Medical Association,* 2007, 298(17):2038-2047.

[9] Hershko C, Camaschella C: How I treat unexplained refractory iron deficiency anemia. *Blood,* 2014, 123(3):326-333.

[10] Pasricha SR, Flecknoe-Brown SC, Allen KJ, Gibson PR, McMahon LP, Olynyk JK, Roger SD, Savoia HF, Tampi R, Thomson AR et al. Diagnosis and management of iron deficiency anaemia: a clinical update. *The Medical journal of Australia,* 2010, 193(9):525-532.

[11] Thomas DW, Hinchliffe RF, Briggs C, Macdougall IC, Littlewood T, Cavill I: Guideline for the laboratory diagnosis of functional iron deficiency. *British journal of haematology,* 2013, 161(5):639-648.

[12] Fishbane S, Miyawaki N: Anemia treatment in chronic kidney disease accompanied by diabetes mellitus or congestive heart failure. *Kidney international,* 2010, 77(3):175-177.

[13] Babitt JL, Lin HY: Molecular mechanisms of hepcidin regulation: implications for the anemia of CKD. *American journal of kidney diseases : the official journal of the National Kidney Foundation,* 2010, 55(4):726-741.

[14] Booth GL, Kapral MK, Fung K, Tu JV: Relation between age and cardiovascular disease in men and women with diabetes compared with non-diabetic people: a population-based retrospective cohort study. *Lancet,* 2006, 368(9529):29-36.

[15] Mehdi U, Toto RD: Anemia, diabetes, and chronic kidney disease. *Diabetes care,* 2009, 32(7):1320-1326.

[16] Chen CX, Li YC, Chan SL, Chan KH: Anaemia and type 2 diabetes: implications from a retrospectively studied primary care case series. *Hong Kong medical journal = Xianggang yi xue za zhi / Hong Kong Academy of Medicine,* 2013, 19(3):214-221.

[17] Ronco C, McCullough P, Anker SD, Anand I, Aspromonte N, Bagshaw SM, Bellomo R, Berl T, Bobek I, Cruz DN et al. Cardio-renal syndromes: report from the consensus conference of the acute dialysis quality initiative. *European heart journal,* 2010, 31(6):703-711.

[18] Pereira CA, Roscani MG, Zanati SG, Matsubara BB: Anemia, heart failure and evidence-based clinical management. *Arq. Bras Cardiol.,* 2013, 101(1):87-92.

[19] Shah R, Agarwal AK: Anemia associated with chronic heart failure: current concepts. *Clinical interventions in aging,* 2013, 8:111-122.

[20] Anker SD, Comin Colet J, Filippatos G, Willenheimer R, Dickstein K, Drexler H, Luscher TF, Bart B, Banasiak W, Niegowska J et al. Ferric carboxymaltose in patients with heart failure and iron deficiency. *The New England journal of medicine,* 2009, 361(25):2436-2448.

[21] Price EA, Mehra R, Holmes TH, Schrier SL: Anemia in older persons: etiology and evaluation. *Blood cells, molecules & diseases,* 2011, 46(2):159-165.

[22] Maccio A, Madeddu C: Management of anemia of inflammation in the elderly. *Anemia,* 2012, 2012:563251.

[23] Landi F, Russo A, Danese P, Liperoti R, Barillaro C, Bernabei R, Onder G: Anemia status, hemoglobin concentration, and mortality in nursing home older residents. *Journal of the American Medical Directors Association,* 2007, 8(5):322-327.

[24] Pang WW, Schrier SL: Anemia in the elderly. *Current opinion in hematology,* 2012, 19(3):133-140.

[25] Joosten E, Ghesquiere B, Linthoudt H, Krekelberghs F, Dejaeger E, Boonen S, Flamaing J, Pelemans W, Hiele M, Gevers AM: Upper and lower gastrointestinal evaluation of elderly inpatients who are iron deficient. *The American journal of medicine,* 1999, 107(1):24-29.

[26] Thorpe SJ, Heath A, Sharp G, Cook J, Ellis R, Worwood M: A WHO reference reagent for the Serum Transferrin Receptor (sTfR): international collaborative study to evaluate a recombinant soluble transferrin receptor preparation. *Clinical chemistry and laboratory medicine : CCLM / FESCC,* 2010, 48(6):815-820.

[27] Lopez-Sierra M, Calderon S, Gomez J, Pilleux L: Prevalence of Anaemia and Evaluation of Transferrin Receptor (sTfR) in the Diagnosis of Iron Deficiency in the Hospitalized Elderly Patients: Anaemia Clinical Studies in Chile. *Anemia,* 2012, 2012:646201.

[28] Goodnough LT, Schrier SL: Evaluation and management of anemia in the elderly. *American journal of hematology,* 2014, 89(1):88-96.

[29] Cancelo-Hidalgo MJ, Castelo-Branco C, Palacios S, Haya-Palazuelos J, Ciria-Recasens M, Manasanch J, Perez-Edo L: Tolerability of different oral iron supplements: a systematic review. *Current medical research and opinion,* 2013, 29(4):291-303.

[30] Ji H, Yardley JH: Iron medication-associated gastric mucosal injury. *Archives of pathology & laboratory medicine,* 2004, 128(7):821-822.

[31] Alleyne M, Horne MK, Miller JL: Individualized treatment for iron-deficiency anemia in adults. *The American journal of medicine,* 2008, 121(11):943-948.

[32] Geisser P, Burckhardt S: The pharmacokinetics and pharmacodynamics of iron preparations. *Pharmaceutics,* 2011, 3(1):12-33.

[33] Ortiz R, Toblli JE, Romero JD, Monterrosa B, Frer C, Macagno E, Breymann C: Efficacy and safety of oral iron(III) polymaltose complex versus ferrous sulfate in pregnant women with iron-deficiency anemia: a multicenter, randomized, controlled study. The journal of maternal-fetal & neonatal medicine : the official journal of the European Association of Perinatal Medicine, the Federation of Asia and Oceania Perinatal

Societies, *the International Society of Perinatal Obstet,* 2011, 24(11):1347-1352.

[34] Yasa B, Agaoglu L, Unuvar E: Efficacy, Tolerability, and Acceptability of Iron Hydroxide Polymaltose Complex versus Ferrous Sulfate: A Randomized Trial in Pediatric Patients with Iron Deficiency Anemia. *International journal of pediatrics,* 2011, 2011:524520.

[35] Nissenson AR, Berns JS, Sakiewicz P, Ghaddar S, Moore GM, Schleicher RB, Seligman PA: Clinical evaluation of heme iron polypeptide: sustaining a response to rHuEPO in hemodialysis patients. *American journal of kidney diseases : the official journal of the National Kidney Foundation,* 2003, 42(2):325-330.

[36] Grasbeck R, Kouvonen I, Lundberg M, Tenhunen R: An intestinal receptor for heme. *Scandinavian journal of haematology,* 1979, 23(1):5-9.

[37] Young MF, Griffin I, Pressman E, McIntyre AW, Cooper E, McNanley T, Harris ZL, Westerman M, O'Brien KO: Utilization of iron from an animal-based iron source is greater than that of ferrous sulfate in pregnant and nonpregnant women. *The Journal of nutrition,* 2010, 140(12):2162-2166.

[38] Nagaraju SP, Cohn A, Akbari A, Davis JL, Zimmerman DL: Heme iron polypeptide for the treatment of iron deficiency anemia in non-dialysis chronic kidney disease patients: a randomized controlled trial. *BMC nephrology,* 2013, 14:64.

[39] Barraclough KA, Brown F, Hawley CM, Leary D, Noble E, Campbell SB, Isbel NM, Mudge DW, van Eps CL, Johnson DW: A randomized controlled trial of oral heme iron polypeptide versus oral iron supplementation for the treatment of anaemia in peritoneal dialysis patients: HEMATOCRIT trial. Nephrology, dialysis, transplantation : official publication of the European Dialysis and Transplant Association - European Renal Association 2012, 27(11):4146-4153.

[40] Macdougall IC, Obrador GT: How important is transfusion avoidance in 2013? Nephrology, dialysis, transplantation : official publication of the European Dialysis and Transplant Association - *European Renal Association,* 2013, 28(5):1092-1099.

[41] Macdougall IC, Fishbane S, Duliege AM: Peginesatide for anemia in chronic kidney disease. *The New England journal of medicine,* 2013, 368(16):1553-1554.

[42] Singh AK, Szczech L, Tang KL, Barnhart H, Sapp S, Wolfson M, Reddan D, Investigators C: Correction of anemia with epoetin alfa in

chronic kidney disease. *The New England journal of medicine,* 2006, 355(20):2085-2098.
[43] Pfeffer MA, Burdmann EA, Chen CY, Cooper ME, de Zeeuw D, Eckardt KU, Feyzi JM, Ivanovich P, Kewalramani R, Levey AS et al. A trial of darbepoetin alfa in type 2 diabetes and chronic kidney disease. *The New England journal of medicine,* 2009, 361(21):2019-2032.
[44] Schiller B, Bhat P, Sharma A: Safety and effectiveness of ferumoxytol in hemodialysis patients at 3 dialysis chains in the United States over a 12-month period. *Clin. Ther.,* 2014, 36(1):70-83.
[45] Locatelli F, Barany P, Covic A, De Francisco A, Del Vecchio L, Goldsmith D, Horl W, London G, Vanholder R, Van Biesen W et al. Kidney Disease: Improving Global Outcomes guidelines on anaemia management in chronic kidney disease: a European Renal Best Practice position statement. Nephrology, dialysis, transplantation : official publication of the European Dialysis and Transplant Association - *European Renal Association,* 2013, 28(6):1346-1359.
[46] Stancu S, Barsan L, Stanciu A, Mircescu G: Can the response to iron therapy be predicted in anemic nondialysis patients with chronic kidney disease? *Clinical journal of the American Society of Nephrology : CJASN,* 2010, 5(3):409-416.
[47] Qunibi WY: The efficacy and safety of current intravenous iron preparations for the management of iron-deficiency anaemia: a review. *Arzneimittel-Forschung,* 2010, 60(6a):399-412.
[48] Vadhan-Raj S, Strauss W, Ford D, Bernard K, Boccia R, Li J, Allen LF: Efficacy and safety of IV ferumoxytol for adults with iron deficiency anemia previously unresponsive to or unable to tolerate oral iron. *American journal of hematology,* 2014, 89(1):7-12.
[49] Lyseng-Williamson KA, Keating GM: Ferric carboxymaltose: a review of its use in iron-deficiency anaemia. *Drugs,* 2009, 69(6):739-756.
[50] Onken JE, Bregman DB, Harrington RA, Morris D, Buerkert J, Hamerski D, Iftikhar H, Mangoo-Karim R, Martin ER, Martinez CO et al. Ferric carboxymaltose in patients with iron-deficiency anemia and impaired renal function: the REPAIR-IDA trial. *Nephrology, dialysis, transplantation : official publication of the European Dialysis and Transplant Association - European Renal Association* 2014, 29(4):833-842.
[51] Qunibi WY, Martinez C, Smith M, Benjamin J, Mangione A, Roger SD: A randomized controlled trial comparing intravenous ferric carboxymaltose with oral iron for treatment of iron deficiency anaemia

of non-dialysis-dependent chronic kidney disease patients. *Nephrology, dialysis, transplantation : official publication of the European Dialysis and Transplant Association - European Renal Association,* 2011, 26(5):1599-1607.

[52] Drueke TB, Parfrey PS: Summary of the KDIGO guideline on anemia and comment: reading between the (guide)line(s). *Kidney international,* 2012, 82(9):952-960.

[53] Vaziri ND: Understanding iron: promoting its safe use in patients with chronic kidney failure treated by hemodialysis. *American journal of kidney diseases : the official journal of the National Kidney Foundation,* 2013, 61(6):992-1000.

[54] Flight MH: Deal watch: AstraZeneca bets on FibroGen's anaemia drug. *Nature reviews Drug discovery,* 2013, 12(10):730.

[55] Swedberg K, Young JB, Anand IS, Cheng S, Desai AS, Diaz R, Maggioni AP, McMurray JJ, O'Connor C, Pfeffer MA et al. Treatment of anemia with darbepoetin alfa in systolic heart failure. *The New England journal of medicine,* 2013, 368(13):1210-1219.

In: Anemia
Editor: Alice Hallman

ISBN: 978-1-63321-775-1
© 2014 Nova Science Publishers, Inc.

Chapter 8

Strategy for Treating Anemia in Chronic Kidney Disease Patients from the Standpoint of Iron Utility

Daisuke Harada[1], Takehisa Kawata[1] and Masaaki Inaba[2]
[1]Nephrology Research Laboratories, Nephrology R & D Unit,
R & D Division, Kyowa Hakko Kirin Co., Ltd., Japan
[2]Department of Endocrinology, Metabolism and Molecular Medicine,
Osaka City University Graduate School of Medicine, Osaka, Japan

Abstract

Anemia is a common complication in patients with chronic kidney disease (CKD). In the past, clinical evidence has accumulated indicating that anemia is associated with higher mortality in CKD patients. Although erythropoiesis-stimulating agents (ESAs) had been considered to contribute to an improved quality of life in CKD patients, recent randomized controlled trials elucidated that high target hemoglobin levels in patients receiving ESAs were associated with an increased risk of cardiovascular events and death, due partly to either erythropoietin resistance or to pre-existing cardiovascular disease (CVD). There are many factors associated with erythropoietin resistance, and inefficient iron utilization has been considered to be one of the main factors. For patients with erythropoietin resistance, it is necessary to increase the dose of intravenous (IV) iron to maintain appropriate levels of transferrin saturation (TSAT). However, excess iron use is followed by resultant increases in either serum ferritin or hepcidin, which are known to be independent factors associated with increased mortality in dialysis patients. Accumulating evidence, including that from the Dialysis Outcomes and Practice Patterns Study, has indicated that a reduction of the IV iron dose by itself, along with the resultant reduction of the serum ferritin or hepcidin levels, might improve the mortality in dialysis patients. Dialysis therapy in Japan has met with greater success than that other countries in terms of the improvement of mortality.

We have recently reported that a long-acting ESA, darbepoetin (DPO)-α, had more potent suppressive effects on the serum hepcidin level than short-acting erythropoietin, and that the serum ferritin level and the dose of IV iron were reduced in the patients on DPO-α to maintain the Hb and TSAT. These data clearly indicate that DPO-α is superior to ESA with regard to improving the iron utility, and thus the life expectancy, in dialysis patients.

1. Renal Anemia and Its Management by Erythropoiesis-Stimulating Agents

Anemia is an expected feature of chronic kidney disease (CKD) once the glomerular filtration rate (GFR) drops below 60 mL/min. Prospective cohort studies suggest that there is a 1% prevalence of anemia for patients with a GFR of 60 mL/min, rising to 9% for those with a GFR below 30 mL/min, and 33-67% for those with a GFR below 15 mL/min [1]. Each 1 g/dL decrease in the mean hemoglobin (Hb) level was independently associated with increases in mortality and cardiac complications in patients with end-stage renal disease (ESRD) [2]. Patients with a hematocrit (Ht) level of <30% have also been shown to have a significantly higher risk of all-cause and cardiac mortality than those with Ht between 30-36% [3].

Severe anemia (Hb < 9g/dL) is highly associated with cardiac complications, such as left ventricular hypertrophy and cardiovascular disease, and leads to an impaired quality of life [4]. Although some randomized controlled trials (RCT) have been performed to examine the hypothesis that increasing the Hb level using erythropoiesis-stimulating agents (ESAs) might lower these risks and improve the quality of life (QOL), three large-scale RCTs (the CHOIR, CREATE and TREAT) failed to demonstrate such beneficial effects of ESA except on fatigue. Instead, in contrast to the expectations, these RCTs demonstrated an increased risk of cardiovascular events and death in the high Hb target patients [5-7].

Three Large-RCTs in Other Countries

CHOIR

The results of the Correction of Hemoglobin in Outcomes and Renal Insufficiency (CHOIR) trial were reported in 2006 [5]. The open-label, randomized, controlled clinical trial enrolled 1,432 patients with anemia and CKD stage 3-5 compared the cardiovascular and renal outcomes for two groups randomized to receive epoetin-α to achieve a mean Hb level of 11.3 g/dL (N=717) versus 13.5 g/dL (N=715). The primary endpoint was the time to the composite of death, myocardial infarction, hospitalization for congestive heart failure or stroke. The secondary outcomes included the time to renal replacement therapy, hospitalization for either cardiovascular causes or any cause and the QOL. Patients were to be followed for approximately three years and the study was powered to show a 25% reduction in the composite event rate in the higher Hb group. All patients were included in the final analysis in an intention to treat model. After three months, a difference in the Hb values between the two groups was observed.

The trial was terminated at the recommendation of the data and safety monitoring board after recording 125 events in the higher Hb group versus 97 events in the lower Hb group (p=0.03). These included deaths, myocardial infarctions, strokes and hospitalizations for congestive heart failure. They concluded that the likelihood of showing a benefit in the higher Hb group was negligible. Although no individual primary outcome reached statistical significance, there appeared to be a trend among the higher Hb group toward an increased rate of hospitalization for chronic heart failure (p=0.07) and death (p=0.07). The QOL scores were similar between the groups.

CREATE

The results of the Cardiovascular Risk Reduction by Early Anemia Treatment with Epoetin Beta trial (CREATE) were also published in 2006 [6]. This RCT was a randomized, controlled clinical trial that enrolled 603 patients to study the cardiovascular benefit of epoetin beta in anemic patients with CKD stages 3 and 4. Patients were randomly assigned to a target Hb in the normal range (13.0-15.0 g/dL, N=301) versus a subnormal level (10.5-11.5 g/dL, N=302). The primary endpoint was a composite of eight cardiovascular events, which included the time to the first cardiovascular event, sudden death, myocardial infarction, acute heart failure, stroke, transient ischemic attack, angina pectoris or cardiac arrhythmia resulting in hospitalization and complications of peripheral vascular disease. The secondary endpoints included death from any cause, death from cardiovascular causes and hospitalization for any cause, among others. The study was powered to detect an annual reduced incidence of the primary endpoint of 15%. At the end of study, the Hb levels between the two groups differed by 1.5 g/dL. Compared to the normal Hb group, the subnormal Hb group did not show significantly more first cardiovascular events or a significantly greater decline in the GFR, but the time to initiation of dialysis after 18 months of the trial was significantly shorter among those treated to obtain a normal Hb (p=0.03). Nevertheless, a total of 105 primary cardiovascular events occurred (58 in the normal Hb group versus 47 in the subnormal Hb group, p=NS). The general health and physical function were significantly improved in the normal target relative to the subnormal target Hb group (p=0.003 and p<0.001, respectively). The investigators concluded that early complete correction of anemia did not reduce the risk of cardiovascular events among anemic patients with CKD stage 3 and 4, although the higher target Hb level did appear to provide some benefits.

TREAT

In 2009, the results of the Trial to Reduce cardiovascular Events with Aranesp Therapy (TREAT) were reported [7]. In the TREAT, 4,038 patients with anemia and diabetic CKD of stages 3 and 4 were enrolled. Randomly assigned patients were treated with darbepoetin-α to achieve an Hb level of approximately 13.0 g/dL (N=2,012), and the remainder of the patients received placebo (N=2,026) and rescue DPO-α therapy if and when the Hb level fell below 9.0 g/dL. The primary endpoints included the composite outcomes of death or cardiovascular events and a composite outcome of the time to death or ESRD. The secondary endpoints included the time to death, death from cardiovascular causes, rate of GFR decline and QOL measures. The trial was powered to detect a 20% reduction in the risk for the primary endpoint among those targeted to obtain a higher Hb level. At the end of the trial, there were no significant differences in the primary cardiovascular composite endpoints. However, a significantly higher proportion of patients suffered fatal or non-fatal strokes among those treated with DPO-α (5% versus 2.6%, p<0.001), despite no evident difference between the blood pressures in the two groups. The renal composite endpoint was reached by 32.4% of the patients in the treatment arm and 30.5% in the placebo arm (p=0.29). A higher proportion of patients in the placebo group required cardiac revascularization (5.8% versus 4.2%, p=0.02). A significantly higher proportion of patients randomized to the placebo arm required transfusions compared to those in the treatment arm (24.5% versus 14.8%, p<0.001).

RCT to Investigate the Renal Protective Effects of the Target Hb Levels in Pre-Dialysis CKD Patients in Japan

As mentioned above, large-scale RCTs to examine the beneficial effects of ESA therapy described no renoprotective effects in a high Hb target group (≥13g/dL) compared with a low Hb target group (9.0-11.5g/dL). Unexpectedly, the high Hb target group tended to have higher cardiovascular risk. These findings offered evidence for the KDIGO recommendation (Grade 1A) that 'ESAs should not be used to intentionally increase the Hb concentration above 13.0 g/dL'. On the other hand, several clinical reports have also suggested that ESA therapy can prevent the progression of renal failure in pre-dialysis CKD patients. The preservation of the renal function by recombinant human erythropoietin (rHuEPO) is reportedly achieved at Hb levels of 11.0-13.0 g/dL, which are higher than the conventional target of approximately 10.0 g/dL [8]. Gouva et al. reported that the renal survival rates might be increased by the early introduction of rHuEPO treatment to increase the Hb levels to 13.0 g/dL compared to those who began rHuEPO treatment at Hb levels < 9.0 g/dL [9]. Nangaku have also suggested that the correction of anemia using an ESA could contribute to renal protection by improving chronic renal tubulointerstitial ischemia [10].

In 2012, it was reported that a three-year RCT had been performed to investigate the renal protective effects at target Hb levels in patients with CKD in Japan [11]. In this study, 321 pre-dialysis anemic CKD patients [Hb < 10 g/dL and serum creatinine (Cr) 2-6 mg/dL at the start of the study] were assigned to one of two groups, a high Hb group (11.0 ≤ Hb < 13.0 g/dL, N=161) treated with long-acting DPO-α or a low Hb group (9.0 ≤ Hb <11.0 g/dL, N=160) treated with short-acting epoetin-α. The primary endpoints were the following events: doubling of the serum Cr concentration, initiation of dialysis, renal transplantation and death. An intergroup comparison of the renal survival rates using a Cox regression model incorporating covariates such as age, sex and the randomization factors of the baseline serum Cr levels, baseline Hb levels and the presence of diabetes as a comorbidity, showed that the hazard ratio (95% CI) for the high Hb group versus the low Hb group was 0.71 (0.52-0.98), indicating that the risk reduction was 29% in the high Hb group. The risk of developing the primary endpoint events was significantly lower (the risk reduction was 29%) in the high Hb group than in the low Hb group (p=0.035).

Cardiovascular events occurred in both the high Hb patients (39.1%) and low Hb patients (37.5%), and the rates did not differ significantly between the two groups of patients. The pre-dialysis CKD patients with higher Hb levels treated with DPO-α maintained a higher renal function, lower left ventricular mass index, and higher QOL scores than those with lower Hb treated with EPO-α, suggesting beneficial effects of higher Hb levels in the pre-dialysis CKD patients [12].

2. The Differences in the Dialysis Outcomes and Practice Patterns Study (DOPPS) among Patients in Japan, Europe and the United States (US)

The DOPPS was an international prospective cohort study of adult hemodialysis (HD) patients from 12 countries (Australia, Belgium, Canada, France, Germany, Italy, Japan, New Zealand, Spain, Sweden, the United Kingdom and the US). The data obtained from the DOPPS are therefore suitable for comparisons of the patients in Japan, Europe and the US. Below, we discuss the differences in the mortality, management of anemia and intravenous (IV) iron use in Japan, Europe and the US.

International Mortality Trends

The mortality rate of dialysis patients has been remarkably lower in Japan than in the other 11 countries, due in part to the high-quality care offered in Japan, including national screening programs for kidney disease, a greater focus on the management of patients with CKD, readily accessible nephrologist care and excellent preparation for dialysis [13-15], as well as the exceptionally high early use of arteriovenous fistulas [16]. For many years, the mortality of patients on dialysis has been higher in the US than in many other countries [17].

In addition to the healthcare, one of the main differences between Japan and other countries is the lower use of IV iron, with a resultant decrease in the serum ferritin level, although the transferrin saturation (TSAT) was maintained at the same level as in other countries [18]. Since it was reported that either the dose of IV iron administered or a high serum ferritin level is significantly associated with a higher mortality rate in HD patients, it is possible that the Renal Anemia Guideline of Japanese Society of Dialysis Therapy (JSDT) prohibiting the use of IV iron in those with a serum ferritin level >100 ng/mL or a TSAT>20% [19] might contribute to the reduction of mortality in Japanese HD patients.

Differences in the Management of Anemia among Countries

The patient mortality rate depends on the management of anemia. Pisoni et al. [20] described that the management of anemia varies across the 12 countries included in the DOPPS, and that the target Hb level is lower in Japan than in the other 11 DOPPS countries, ranging from 11.1 g/dL in France to 12.0 g/dL in Sweden. This study reported significantly higher use of IV iron, ranging from administration to 53% of the patient in Italy to 89% in Belgium, compared to 38% of the patients in Japan. Furthermore, Japan has the highest rate of using a native arteriovenous fistula and the lowest use of central venous catheters among all of the countries in the DOPPS. Since catheter use, which is common in the other 11 countries, is known to be strongly associated with the risk of infection and inflammation [21], the resultant inflammation might increase the serum hepcidin level and decrease the iron utility by increasing the serum IL-6 levels [22]. As partial confirmation of this relationship, an evaluation of the DOPPS Phase 2 data revealed a much lower occurrence of septicemia among HD patients in Japan compared to those in the other DOPPS countries. This might increase the need for IV iron to maintain the TSAT by decreasing the iron utility, resulting in lower Hb levels [20]

Differences in IV Iron Use

IV iron has been increasingly prescribed for dialysis patients [23] after the dose of ESA has been restricted to avoid the dangers associated with its overuse [24]. In response to the FDA ESA label change in 2010, the DOPPS Practice Monitor for US dialysis care reported that the percentage of dialysis patients receiving IV iron increased from 57% to 71% between 2010 and 2011 [23]. Fuller et al. also reported that the US monthly IV iron use rose from 55%

to 68% between 2010 and 2012 [24], while it was unchanged in Europe and Japan. On the basis of the DOPPS cohort studied between 1999 and 2011, Bailie et al. [18] reported that (i) there is large variability internationally and over time in all facets of prescription practices, including the choice of IV iron product, choice of IV iron dose and frequency of administration, (ii) there is much lower use of IV iron in Japan, and (iii) Japan had the lowest serum ferritin, but a similar TSAT level, among the 12 countries. Furthermore, between 2010 and 2012, the mean ferritin level rose by 35% to 825 ng/mL in the US and by 8% to 514 ng/mL in European countries, while there was no significant increase during the same period in Japan [25].

Relationship between Iron and Mortality

According to the DOPPS Phase 4 data [18], the US and some Europe countries had serum ferritin levels over 500 ng/mL with a percentage IV iron use ranging from 70% to 90%. On the other hand, the mean serum ferritin level was about 200 ng/mL [25], and the utilization of IV iron remains at around 40% in Japan. Since the TSAT around 25% in Japan did not differ significantly from those in the US and Europe, this suggested that the iron utility might be better in Japan than in other countries. Since the dose of IV iron was significantly and positively correlated with the serum ferritin level, but not with the TSAT, it is possible that the overuse of IV iron might increase oxidative stress without increasing the dose of iron available for erythropoiesis [26]. Therefore, an increase in the serum ferritin level might reflect iron overload.

In a study of HD patients receiving ESA and IV iron, the iron storage in the liver detected by MRI increased with the increasing dose of IV iron [27]. It has been shown that higher serum ferritin levels resulting from higher doses of IV iron could worsen the prognosis for patients. Hasuike et al. reported that a serum ferritin level ≥100 ng/mL was significantly associated with a poorer prognosis compared to a serum ferritin level < 100 ng/mL in 90 Japanese HD patients [28]. Bailie et al. [29] also reported that there were associations between an increased dose of IV iron and increased mortality based on the DOPPS Phase 2 and 3 data. Compared to HD patients receiving IV iron at doses between 100-199 mg/month, those with an average dose of IV iron ≥400 mg/month had a 21% higher risk of all-cause mortality and a 41% higher risk of cardiovascular-related mortality. It was also reported that the serum ferritin level might be one of the strongest predictors of the progression of atherosclerosis [30].

3. Iron and Its Use for Chronic Renal Failure

Iron Metabolism

There is 3-4 g of iron present in the human body. About 2 g of this iron is present mainly as heme in hemoglobin inside erythroid cells or as myoglobin inside muscles. Macrophages in the spleen, liver and bone marrow keep transient fractions of iron. Since excess free iron becomes harmful for cells due to the production of oxygen radicals by the Fenton reaction, it is stored as ferritin in the liver. The iron concentrations in the serum remain stable up to 10-30µM. Since the capacity for iron excretion from the body is only 1-2 mg/day, and occurs only through the desquamation of epithelial cells in the intestine [31-33], the iron excretion cannot be increased, and thus, the excessive iron resulting from IV iron is only stored as ferritin within cells [31, 32].

Iron is transported through the cell membrane by an iron transporter, ferroportin. Since the activity of ferroportin is strictly regulated by the iron regulatory hormone, known as hepcidin, it is the most important factor that regulates iron trafficking [34]. Hepcidin binds to ferroportin on the plasma membrane of various cells, promoting its internalization, and resulting in its degradation. Hepcidin synthesis is stimulated by the extracellular and intracellular iron concentrations through the activation of bone morphogenetic protein receptors, resulting in a decrease in the distribution of iron into the circulation. Therefore hepcidin-induced inactivation of ferroportin causes intracellular iron retention [35]. Because hepcidin-mediated iron redistribution has a role in the host defense, hepcidin production is also upregulated by inflammation [36]. Increased hepcidin concentrations in plasma are pathogenic in patients with anemia associated with inflammation.

Iron Overload and Tissue Damage, including Kidney Damage

Excess iron poses a threat to cells and tissues because of its ability to catalyze the generation of reactive radicals, which is intimately involved in a variety of complications. Accordingly, it was previously reported that a high serum ferritin level might be associated with hospitalization, morbidity and all-cause mortality in HD patients [37]. It was suggested that iron, which preferentially accumulates in macrophages, especially those in ruptured human atherosclerotic lesions, accelerates the atherosclerotic changes to the ruptured atherosclerotic plaques by causing local oxidative stress [38]. In fact, it was reported that high levels of serum ferritin adversely affect the risk of ischemic heart and increase the mortality rate [39, 40]. These background data clearly indicate that the excessive accumulation of iron in body stores might have harmful effects due to the increased oxidative stress.

Iron overload also injures renal tubular cells and reduces the kidney function [41]. Excess iron above the capacity of the iron saturation of transferrin can be present as non-transferrin-bound iron in the serum. This iron might be filtered through the glomerulus, which may then reach the renal tubule epithelial cells and cause injury. Mice fed an iron-enriched diet showed renal tubular damage and subsequent renal failure. Patients with transfusion-related iron overload also showed renal tubule dysfunction. These findings demonstrated that there was iron accumulation in renal tubular cells, and that this caused severe renal tubular damage, which was associated with a worsening of renal failure in patients with CRF. Since excess iron administration induces the expression of hepcidin, thereby causing iron trapping along the entire nephron, it might worsen renal failure.

IV Iron Use for CRF

As mentioned above, the excessive use of IV iron may result in undesirable patient outcomes. The threshold for iron toxicity is unclear, although Vaziri et al. reported that iron use in patients with CKD is beneficial and safe up to a serum ferritin level around 300-500 ng/mL [42]. A retrospective analysis suggested that serum ferritin levels from 500-1200 ng/mL are safe [43]. The Dialysis Patients' Response to Intravenous Iron with Elevated Ferritin (DRIVE) I and DRIVE II trials investigated liberal IV iron use in HD patients [44, 45]. In those studies, the ferric gluconate given dialysis patients was effective for improving the anemia of HD patients who had ferritin levels up to 1200 ng/mL and a TSAT under 25%. These trials suggested that there were no adverse effects of IV iron even for patients with high plasma ferritin levels but a relatively low TSAT. However, since this observation period was only 12 weeks, the potential risks of the excessive use of IV iron compounds over a longer period have not been sufficiently examined.

HD patients lose 1.5-3.0 g of iron yearly due to blood losses during HD sessions. In the DRIVE study, since at least 1.0 g iron was administered for only 12 weeks, it is likely that there was no iron overload, because overload occurs only when such a high dose of iron continues to be administered for a long time. Canavese et al. found that iron overload occurs in as many as 70% of dialysis patients treated with IV iron, although the majority of this dialysis population had serum ferritin levels below 500 ng/mL [37]. It was suggested that the hepatic iron content correlated with the serum ferritin level, and that a serum ferritin level > 340 ng/mL coincides with iron overload detected by MRI. Ferrari et al. have shown a drastic increase in the hepatic iron content in HD patients receiving standard IV iron therapy, which is the same level administered to hemochromatosis patients [46]. Rostocker et al. also indicated that iron overload is common in ESRD patients treated with a standard IV iron regimen [27].

In CKD patients with systemic inflammation, who are often hyporesponsive or even resistant to ESA and/or iron therapy, care should be taken when the use of high doses of IV iron preparations is considered. Anemia in CKD patients with systemic inflammation should be treated without IV iron. High ferritin and hepcidin levels in CKD patients with systemic inflammation may represent a biological "red light" for IV iron therapy, which should be addressed in order to not only prevent iron overload and amplification of the inflammation, but also prevent the production of reactive oxygen species, well-known mediators of tissue damage.

No information has been obtained on the long-term safety of prescribing IV iron therapy to dialysis patients with a serum ferritin level >500 ng/mL. The European Renal Best Practice (ERBP) position statement recommends that a TSAT value ≤50% and a serum ferritin level ≤500 ng/mL should be maintained in patients on dialysis. In pre-dialysis CKD patients, the TSAT value should be restricted more strictly under 30% [47]. The DOPPS Practice Monitor showed that IV iron administration is discontinued until the ferritin value exceeds 800 ng/mL in most facilities, and that 25% of surveyed facilities had serum ferritin levels exceeding 800 ng/mL in the majority of their patients [48].

In contrast, the range of ferritin values considered to require caution is quite different in Japan. In the Nishinomiya Study [28], in which 90HD patients were monitored for the influence of serum ferritin on the survival rates during a study period of 107 months, it was demonstrated that a serum ferritin level >100 ng/mL was associated with a significantly poorer prognosis in a Kaplan-Meier analysis. This study provided evidence for the renal anemia guidelines of the JSDT that the serum ferritin level should be kept at ≤100 ng/mL to reduce the mortality rate in HD patients.

The Impact of a Long-Acting Erythropoiesis-Stimulating Agent on the Iron Metabolism

Shimizu et al. have reported that a long-acting ESA, DPO-α, potently suppressed the hepcidin mRNA levels from days 1 to 4 when erythropoiesis had been induced [49]. The serum iron level and TSAT decreased from days 1 to 4 after DPO-α administration, in response to the increased iron demand for activated erythropoiesis. We have demonstrated a greater effect for DPO-α in the suppression of serum hepcidin, and thus increased utility of iron for erythropoiesis in HD patients [50]. In this long-term crossover study, DPO-α decreased the serum ferritin and hepcidin levels further after changing from a short-acting ESA, rHuEPO, while it maintained the Hb level within the same target level of 10.0-11.0 g/dL.

Since there was no significant change in the Hb level, the serum iron level or the TSAT throughout the study between two ESAs, the data suggested that DPO-α did not decrease the amount of iron utilizable for erythropoiesis in spite of the decreased body iron stores indicated by the reduced serum ferritin level. These data clearly demonstrated that DPO-α might improve the efficacy of iron utilization for erythropoiesis in HD patients. The reduction in the serum ferritin level during the DPO-α treatment might have resulted from the decreased dose of IV iron administered based on the Japanese renal anemia guidelines, in which a TSAT >20% was the cut-off value to prohibit IV iron administration.

Because the long-acting DPO-α suppressed the serum hepcidin production more potently than the short-acting rHuEPO, iron seemed to be mobilized from iron stores in the form of ferritin into the circulation, and finally into the bone marrow for erythropoiesis. It was recently reported that erythroferrone, a member of the TNF-α family, is secreted from erythroblasts, and is the main factor involved in the suppression of serum hepcidin during the process of stimulated erythropoiesis [51]. Therefore, it is possible that the more potent erythropoiesis induced by DPO-α was substantiated by the greater utility of iron by an increased level of erythroferrone, since the continuing entry of iron is needed to maintain stimulated erythropoiesis because stimulated erythropoiesis requires the additional entry of a huge amount of iron into the bone marrow.

As a result, the iron stores in the body's cells are reduced with DPO-α treatment, as represented by the reduced serum ferritin level, although the serum iron available for erythropoiesis was maintained at the same level, as reflected by the unchanged TSAT levels.

It has been suggested that the long-acting ESA, DPO-α, causes efficient erythropoiesis because it results in better utilization of iron in the bone marrow from body stores to induce erythropoiesis effectively, and thus could allow the IV iron to be restricted to maintain lower levels of serum ferritin, which would protect cells against the possible harmful effects of excessive iron. This might offer evidence of the advantage of using long-acting DPO-α as the primary therapeutic agent for renal anemia in HD patients, compared to the short-acting rHuEPO.

Conclusion

Caution is required to interpret the safety of iron administration correctly, since iron administration has been proved to be safe by large clinical studies. However, there have been no clinical studies which have shown the safety of iron administration for a long period. In the DOPPS data, it was found that Japanese patients being treated with dialysis had a remarkably better prognosis compared with that of Westerners. It seems that the lower amount of iron used in Japan may contribute to this better prognosis. The best regimen of iron administration will need to be established after taking into consideration the accumulation of iron inside the body.

Although various clinical studies in countries outside of Japan had shown that the long-term use of DPO-α led to poorer outcomes in terms of heart failure and the general prognosis, a protective effect of DPO-α on the renal function was shown in Japan. It was also reported that DPO-α could improve the iron utilization in red blood cells, reduce the hepcidin level and improve the iron metabolism in dialysis patients [50]. Therefore, the clinical use of a sufficient balance of iron and a long-acting ESA should be recommended. If a long-acting ESA contributes to improving the prognosis, it should be used from an early stage, and guidelines for the use of the agent for target populations should be established.

References

[1] Astor, B. C., Arnett, D. K., Brown, A. et al. (2004). Association of kidney function and hemoglobin with left ventricular morphology among African Americans: the Atherosclerosis Risk in Communities (ARIC) study. *Am J Kidney Dis.*, *43*, 836-45.

[2] Foley, R. N., Parfrey, P. S., Harnett, J. D. et al. (1996). The impact of anemia on cardiomyopathy, morbidity, and and mortality in end-stage renal disease. *Am J Kidney Dis.*, *28*, 53-61.

[3] Ma, J. Z., Ebben, J., Xia, H. et al. (1999). Hematocrit level and associated mortality in hemodialysis patients. *J Am Soc Nephrol.*, *10*, 610-9.

[4] Levin, A., Thompson, C. R., Ethier, J. et al. (1999) Left ventricular mass index increase in early renal disease: impact of decline in hemoglobin. *Am J Kidney Dis.*, *34*, 125-34.

[5] Singh, A. K., Szczech, L., Tang, K. L. et al. (2006). Correction of anemia with epoetin alfa in chronic kidney disease. *N. Engl. J. Med.*, *355*, 2085-98.

[6] Drüeke, T. B., Locatelli, F., Clyne, N. et al. (2006). Normalization of hemoglobin level in patients with chronic kidney disease and anemia. *N. Engl. J. Med.*, *355*, 2071-84.

[7] Pfeffer, M. A., Burdmann, E. A., Chen, C. Y. et al. (2009). A trial of darbepoetin alfa in type 2 diabetes and chronic kidney disease. *N Engl J Med.*, *361*, 2019-32.

[8] Kuriyama, S., Tomonari, H., Yoshida, H. et al. (1997). Reversal of anemia by erythropoietin therapy retards the progression of chronic renal failure, especially in nondiabetic patients. *Nephron*, *77*, 176-85.

[9] Gouva, C., Nikolopoulos, P., Ioannidis, J. P. et al. (2004). Treating anemia early in renal failure patients slows the decline of renal function: a randomized controlled trial. *Kidney Int.*, *66*, 753-60.

[10] Nangaku, M. (2006). Chronic hypoxia and tubulointerstitial injury: a final common pathway to end-stage renal failure. *J Am Soc Nephrol.*, *17*, 17-25.

[11] Tsubakihara, Y., Gejyo, F., Nishi, S. et al. (2012). High target hemoglobin with erythropoiesis-stimulating agents has advantages in the renal function of non-dialysis chronic kidney disease patients. *Ther Apher Dial.*, *16*, 529-40.
[12] Akaishi, M., Hiroe, M., Hada, Y. et al. (2013). Effect of anemia correction on left ventricular hypertrophy in patients with modestly high hemoglobin level and chronic kidney disease. *J Cardiol.*, *62*, 249-56.
[13] Yamagata, K., Nakai, S., Masakane, I. et al. (2012). Ideal timing and predialysis nephrology care duration for dialysis initiation: from analysis of Japanese dialysis initiation survey. *Ther Apher Dial.*, *16*, 54-62.
[14] Yamagata, K., Iseki, K., Nitta, K. et al. (2008). Chronic kidney disease perspectives in Japan and the importance of urinalysis screening. *Clin Exp Nephrol*, *12*, 1-8.
[15] Ando, Y., Ito, S., Uemura, O. et al. (2009). CKD Clinical Practice Guidebook. The essence of treatment for CKD patients. *Clin Exp Nephrol*, *13*, 191-248.
[16] Ethier, J., Mendelssohn, D. C., Elder, S.J. et al. (2008). Vascular access use and outcomes: an international perspective from the Dialysis Outcomes and Practice Patterns Study. *Nephrol Dial Transplant*, *23*, 3219-26.
[17] Goodkin, D. A., Bragg-Gresham, J. L., Koenig, K. G. et al. (2003). Association of comorbid conditions and mortality in hemodialysis patients in Europe, Japan, and the United States in the Dialysis Outcomes and Practice Patterns Study (DOPPS). *J Am Soc Nephrol*, *14*, 3270-7.
[18] Bailie, G. R., Larkina, M., Goodkin, D. A. et al. (2013). Variation in intravenous iron use internationally and over time: the Dialysis Outcomes and Practice Patterns Study (DOPPS). *Nephrol Dial Transplant*, *28*, 2570-9.
[19] Tsubakihara, Y., Nishi, S., Akiba, T. et al. (2010). Japanese Society for Dialysis Therapy: guidelines for renal anemia in chronic kidney disease. *Ther Apher Dial*, *14*, 240-75.
[20] Pisoni, R. L., Bragg-Gresham, J. L., Young, E. W. et al. (2004). Anemia management and outcomes from 12 countries in the Dialysis Outcomes and Practice Patterns Study (DOPPS). *Am J Kidney Dis.*, *44*, 94-111.
[21] Combe, C. H., Pisoni, R. L., Port, F. K. et al. (2001). Dialysis outcomes and practice patterns study: donn´ees sur l'utilisation des cath´eters veineux centraux en hemodialyse chronique. *Nephrologie*, *22*, 379-84.

[22] D'Angelo, G. (2013). Role of hepcidin in the pathophysiology and diagnosis of anemia. *Blood Res.*, *48*, 10-5.
[23] Pisoni, R. L., Fuller, D. S., Bieber, B. A. et al. (2012). The DOPPS practice monitor for US dialysis care: trends through August 2011. *Am. J. Kidney Dis.*, *60*, 160-5.
[24] Iglehart, J. K. (2011). Bundled payment for ESRD - including ESAs in Medicare's dialysis package. *N. Engl. J. Med.*, *364*, 593-5.
[25] Fuller, D. S., Robinson, B. M., Bieber, B. et al. International Comparisons Illustrate Effect of Payment and Regulatory Changes on Anemia Practice in U.S. Hemodialysis Patients: The Dialysis Outcomes and Practice Patterns Study. American Society of Nephrology Renal Week 2013.
[26] Kuo, K. L., Hung, S. C., Lin, Y. P. et al. (2012). Intravenous ferric chloride hexahydrate supplementation induced endothelial dysfunction and increased cardiovascular risk among hemodialysis patients. *PLoS One*, *7*, e50295.
[27] Rostoker, G., Griuncelli, M., Loridon, C. et al. (2012). Hemodialysis-associated hemosiderosis in the era of erythropoiesis-stimulating agents: a MRI study. *Am J Med.*, *125*, 991-9.
[28] Hasuike, Y., Nonoguchi, H., Tokuyama, M. et al. (2010). Serum ferritin predicts prognosis in hemodialysis patients: the Nishinomiya study. *Clin Exp Nephrol.*, *14*, 349-55.
[29] Bailie, G. R., Tong, L., Li, Y., Mason, N. A. et al. Association of Intravenous Iron (ivFe) Dosing with Mortality: Findings from the DOPPS. American Society of Nephrology Renal Week 2010.
[30] Kiechl, S., Willeit, J., Egger, G. et al. (1997). Body iron stores and the risk of carotid atherosclerosis: prospective results from the Bruneck study. *Circulation*, *18*, 3300-7.
[31] Wang, J., Pantopoulos, K. (2011). Biochem J. Regulation of cellular iron metabolism. *Biochem J.*, *434*, 365-81.
[32] Hentze, M. W., Muckenthaler, M. U., Galy, B. et al. (2010). Two to tango: regulation of Mammalian iron metabolism. *Cell*, *142*, 24-38.
[33] Pantopoulos, K., Porwal, S. K., Tartakoff, A. et al. (2012). Biochemistry. *Mechanisms of mammalian iron homeostasis*, *51*, 5705-24.
[34] Ruchala, P. & Nemeth, E. (2014). The pathophysiology and pharmacology of hepcidin. *Trends Pharmacol Sci.*, *35*, 155-61.
[35] Brasse-Lagnel, C., Karim, Z., Letteron, P. et al. (2011). Beaumont C Intestinal DMT1 cotransporter is down-regulated by hepcidin via

proteasome internalization and degradation. *Gastroenterology, 140*, 1261-71.
[36] Ganz, T. & Nemeth, E. (2011). Hepcidin and disorders of iron metabolism. *Annu Rev Med., 62*, 347-60.
[37] Canavese, C., Bergamo, D., Ciccone, G. et al. (2004). Validation of serum ferritin values by magnetic susceptometry in predicting iron overload in dialysis patients. *Kidney Int., 65*, 1091-8.
[38] Stadler, N., Lindner, R. A. & Davies, M. J. (2004). Direct detection and quantification of transition metal ions in human atherosclerotic plaques: evidence for the presence of elevated levels of iron and copper. *Arterioscler Thromb Vasc Biol., 24*, 949-54.
[39] Zhou, Y., Liu, T., Tian, C. et al. (2012). Association of serum ferritin with coronary artery disease. *Clin Biochem., 45*, 1336-41.
[40] Holay, M. P., Choudhary, A. A. & Suryawanshi, S. D. (2012). Serum ferritin-a novel risk factor in acute myocardial infarction. *Indian Heart J., 64*, 173-7.
[41] Martines, A. M., Masereeuw, R., Tjalsma, H. et al. (2013). Iron metabolism in the pathogenesis of iron-induced kidney injury. *Nat Rev Nephrol., 9*, 385-98.
[42] Vaziri, N. D. (2013). Understanding iron: promoting its safe use in patients with chronic kidney failure treated by hemodialysis. *Am J Kidney Dis., 61*, 992-1000.
[43] Kalantar-Zadeh, K., Kalantar-Zadeh, K. & Lee, G. H. (2013). The fascinating but deceptive ferritin: to measure it or not to measure it in chronic kidney disease? *Clin J Am Soc Nephrol.*, Suppl 1: S9-18.
[44] Coyne, D. W., Kapoian, T., Suki, W. et al. (2007). Ferric gluconate is highly efficacious in anemic hemodialysis patients with high serum ferritin and low transferrin saturation: results of the Dialysis Patients' Response to IV Iron with Elevated Ferritin (DRIVE) Study. DRIVE Study Group. *J Am Soc Nephrol., 18*, 975-84.
[45] Kapoian, T., O'Mara, N. B., Singh, A. K. et al. (2008). Ferric gluconate reduces epoetin requirements in hemodialysis patients with elevated ferritin. *J Am Soc Nephrol., 19*, 372-9.
[46] Ferrari, P., Kulkarni, H., Dheda, S. et al. (2011). Serum iron markers are inadequate for guiding iron repletion in chronic kidney disease. *Clin J Am Soc Nephrol., 6*, 77-83.
[47] Goldsmith, D. J., Covic, A., Fouque, D. et al. (2011). Endorsement of the Kidney Disease Improving Global Outcomes (KDIGO) Chronic Kidney Disease-Mineral and Bone Disorder (CKD-MBD) Guidelines: a

European Renal Best Practice (ERBP) commentary statement. *Nephrol Dial Transplant.*, *25*, 3823-31.

[48] Weiner, D. E. & Winkelmayer, W. C. (2013). Commentary on 'The DOPPS practice monitor for U.S. dialysis care: update on trends in anemia management 2 years into the bundle': iron(y) abounds 2 years later. Am *J Kidney Dis.*, *62*, 1217-20.

[49] Simizu, K., Haruyama, W., Ogasawara, Y. et al. (2013). Comparison of erythropoiesis-stimulating activity between Darbepoietin Alfa (DA) and Epoetin beta pegol (C. E. R. A.) in normal rats. *Kidney and Dialysis, 75*, 437-42.

[50] Shoji, S., Inaba, M., Tomosugi, N. et al. (2013). Greater potency of darbepoetin-α than erythropoietin in suppression of serum hepcidin-25 and utilization of iron for erythropoiesis in hemodialysis patients. *Eur J Haematol, 90*, 237-44.

[51] Kautz, L., Jung, G., Valore, E. et al. (2014). Identification of erythroferrone as an erythroid regulator of iron metabolism. *Nat Genet.*, doi:10.1038/ng.2996

In: Anemia
Editor: Alice Hallman

ISBN: 978-1-63321-775-1
© 2014 Nova Science Publishers, Inc.

Chapter 9

Parasitic Anemia: Prevalence, Risk and Management

Somsri Wiwanitkit[1] and Viroj Wiwanitkit[2]
[1]Wiwanitkit House, Bangkhae, Bangkok Thailand
[2]Hainan Medical University, China,
Faculty of Medicine, University of Nis, Serbia

Abstract

Anemia is a common hematological problem that can be seen worldwide and it is still under consideration for global public health. There are many causes of anemia. An important cause is the parasitic infestation. The parasitic anemia can be seen worldwide and this is still the problem in many countries, especially for those in tropical zone. There are many parasites that can induce anemia. In this short article, the authors will summarize and discuss on important kinds of parasitic anemia focusing on prevalence, risk and management.

Keywords: Anemia, risk, parasite

Introduction [1-2]

Anemia is a condition that one has low hemoglobin level. Since hemoglobin is an important biopigment having the role in oxygen carriage and transportation, the low abnormal hemoglobin level can be problematic for human beings. Anemia is a common hematological problem that can be seen worldwide and it is still under consideration for global public health. There are many causes of anemia such as nutritional deficiencies (iron, vitamin B12, folate, etc). An important cause is the parasitic infestation. The parasitic anemia can be seen worldwide and this is still the problem in many countries, especially for those in tropical zone. There are many parasites that can induce anemia. In this short article, the authors will summarize and discuss on important kinds of parasitic anemia focusing on prevalence, risk and management.

Important Parasitic Anemia

1. Hookworm Anemia [3 – 4]

Hookworm is an important nematode that can be seen worldwide and it is common in tropical zone. This worm can infest human by direct penetrating into the foot of human. The problem is usually due to lack of proper toilet usage and lack of shoe wearing. The hookworm lives in the intestine of human and it can reproduce to form the egg. The egg will be passed thorough defecation and can contaminate into the soil. This can be the cycle of infection.

Hookworm has its hooklet that hooks to the human intestine and this cause chronic blood loss. Hence, it is no doubt that chronic hookworm infestation can result in anemia. The anemia due to hookworm infestation is classified into the form of microcytic anemia. This is another common cause of iron deficiency anemia adding to poor intake of iron [5]. The high prevalence of hookworm infestation can be seen in tropical zone especially in the area with poor sanitation. The risks include poor toileting and no wearing shoes. For diagnosis, the anemic patient can be diagnosed to have hookworm infestation by detection of hookworm egg from stool examination. The standard treatment for the hookworm anemia includes a) correction of anemic problem, which is usually by iron supplementation and b) getting rid of hookworm by antiparasitic drug. Smith and Brooker noted that "anemia is most strongly associated with moderate and heavy hookworm infection [6]" and "the impact of anthelmintic treatment is greatest when albendazole is co-administered with praziquantel [6]." The future hope is the development of hookworm vaccine, which is still on its study process [7 – 8].

2. Malarial anemia [9 - 10]

Malaria is an important blood parasitic infection. The malarial parasite directly attacks the red blood cell and cause red blood cell pathology. Hence, it is no doubt that anemia can be seen in malaria and it is called malarial anemia. The anemia due to hookworm infestation is classified into the form of normocytic anemia. Pradhan noted that the nitric oxide produced by parasite is an important cause of anemia [11].

The high prevalence of malaria can be seen in tropical zone especially in the area with abundance of mosquito vector. The risks include exposure to malarial vector. Douglas et al. noted that the problem could be serious in pediatric population [12]. For diagnosis, the anemic patient can be diagnosed to have malaria by detection of parasite within blood smear. The standard treatment for the malarial anemia includes a) correction of anemic problem and b) getting rid of malaria by antimalarial drug.

3. Diphyllobothrial anemia [13]

Diphyllobothrium latum is an important intestinal parasite. This parasite is a tapeworm and can be seen in fish. This cestode infestation can result in anemia, which is in the form of macrocytic anemia [14]. It is accepted as an important cause of pernicious among the Scandinavian [15 – 17]. Intake of uncooked or poorly cooked fish is the risk for getting infestation. For diagnosis, the anemic patient can be diagnosed to have this parasitic infestation by detection of parasitic egg or proglottid by stool examination. The standard treatment for the malarial anemia includes a) correction of anemic problem and b) getting rid of malaria by antimalarial drug. Control of fish and fish product quality is the recommendation for prevention of this fish-borne disease [18].

Conclusion

There are many parasitic diseases that can causes anemia. The anemia resulted from parasitic diseases can be seen in many forms (micro-, normo- or macrocytic forms). The practitioner has to take concern on the possible parasitic causes of anemia in any cases.

References

[1] ANEMIA, a review of its causes and therapy. *Med Times.* 1947 Nov, 75(11), 335-50.
[2] Marriott, HL. A Review of Anæmia. *Postgrad Med J.* 1934 Jul, 10(105), 236-41.
[3] Roche, M; Layrisse, M. The nature and causes of "hookworm anemia". *Am J Trop Med Hyg.* 1966 Nov, 15(6), 1029-102.
[4] Iron deficiency anemia due to hookworm infection in man. *Nutr Rev.* 1968 Feb, 26(2), 47-9.
[5] Miller, JL. Iron deficiency anemia: a common and curable disease. *Cold Spring Harb Perspect Med.* 2013 Jul 1, 3(7). pii: a011866.
[6] Smith, JL; Brooker, S. Impact of hookworm infection and deworming on anaemia in non-pregnant populations: a systematic review. *Trop Med Int Health.* 2010 Jul, 15(7), 776-95.
[7] Hotez, PJ; Bethony, JM; Diemert, DJ; Pearson, M; Loukas, A. Developing vaccines to combat hookworm infection and intestinal schistosomiasis. *Nat Rev Microbiol.* 2010 Nov, 8(11), 814-26.
[8] Diemert, DJ; Bethony, JM; Hotez, PJ. Hookworm vaccines. *Clin Infect Dis.* 2008 Jan 15, 46(2), 282-8.
[9] Gilles, HM. Malaria. *Trop Dis Bull.* 1971 Mar, 68(3), 265-74.
[10] Gilles, HM. Malaria. *Trop Dis Bull.* 1968 Mar, 65(3), 213-8.
[11] Pradhan, P. Malarial anaemia and nitric oxide induced megaloblastic anaemia: a review on the causes of malarial anaemia. *J Vector Borne Dis.* 2009 Jun, 46(2), 100-8.
[12] Douglas, NM; Anstey, NM/ Buffet, PA; Poespoprodjo, JR; Yeo, TW; White, NJ; Price, RN. The anaemia of Plasmodium vivax malaria. *Malar J.* 2012 Apr 27, 11, 135.
[13] Georgi, JR. Tapeworms. *Vet Clin North Am Small Anim Pract.* 1987 Nov, 17(6), 1285-305.

[14] Donoso-Scroppo, M; Raposo, L; Reyes, H; Godorecci, S; Castillo, G. Megaloblastic anemia secondary to infection by Diphyllobothrium latum. *Rev Med Chil.* 1986 Dec, 114(12), 1171-4.

[15] von Bonsdorff, B. Diphyllobothrium latum and pernicious anemia. *Acta Haematol.* 1953 Sep, 10(3), 129-43.

[16] von Bonsdorff, B. Diphyllobothrium latum as a cause of pernicious anemia. *Exp Parasitol.* 1956 Mar, 5(2), 207-30.

[17] von Bonsdorff, B. Pernicious anemia caused by Diphyllobothrium latum, in the light of recent investigations. *Blood.* 1948 Jan, 3(1), 91-102.

[18] Esteban, JG; Muñoz-Antoli, C; Borras, M; Colomina, J; Toledo, R. Human infection by a "fish tapeworm", Diphyllobothrium latum, in a non-endemic country. *Infection.* 2014 Feb, 42(1), 191-4.

Index

A

acetaminophen, 54
acid, 10, 31, 38, 50, 57, 68, 74
acute leukemia, 89
acute myelogenous leukemia, 121
acute myeloid leukemia, 32, 67, 78, 92, 94
adenosine, 23, 59
adenosine phosphate, 23
adhesion, 50
adipose tissue, 44
adolescents, 56, 58, 62
ADP, 10
adulthood, 21, 101
adults, xi, 36, 46, 99, 101, 113, 115, 124, 127, 131, 143, 145
adverse effects, 56, 82, 139, 157
adverse event, 8, 9, 11, 101, 104, 135
Africa, ix, 49, 51, 52, 126
African-American(s), ix, 49, 52, 133
age, ix, xi, 4, 21, 59, 66, 67, 68, 75, 81, 83, 84, 99, 101, 121, 124, 126, 128, 131, 132, 142, 151, 160
ageing population, 125, 140
aggregation, 10, 17
albumin, 26
alcoholic cirrhosis, 41, 46
aldosterone, 3
alpha-tocopherol, 56, 61
amino acid(s), 50, 55, 84, 129

ancestors, ix, 49, 51
androgen, 117
angina, 150
angiogenesis, 4, 44
annotation, 91
annual rate, 42
antibody, 83
antigen, 90, 127
anti-inflammatory drugs, 54
antioxidant(s), vii, viii, 20, 22, 24, 26, 28, 29, 30, 31, 32, 55, 56, 57, 62
antioxidative activity, 24
aplasia, 53
aplastic anemia, 83
apoptosis, 44, 72, 73, 75, 90, 139
appendicular skeleton, 42
Argentina, 65
artery, 2, 14
ascorbic acid, 55, 56, 61
Asia, 126, 143
aspirate, 15, 67, 68, 69, 134
assessment, viii, 14, 20, 22, 63, 68, 79, 102, 106, 108, 113, 119
asymptomatic, ix, 10, 11, 66
atherosclerosis, 117, 155, 162
atherosclerotic plaque, 156, 163
athletes, xi, 100, 105, 106, 111, 114
atomic nucleus, 20
atrial fibrillation, 6
avascular necrosis, 51

B

bacteremia, 54
bacterial infection, 53
Belgium, 152, 153
beneficial effect, 148, 151, 152
benefits, 121, 150
beriberi, 7, 14
bias, 103, 107
bicuspid, 6
bilirubin, 9
biological systems, 32
biomarkers, 46
biopsy, 67, 68
biosynthesis, 22
birth weight, 124
births, ix, 49, 52
bleeding, 4, 6, 11, 13, 15, 69, 100, 101, 129, 133
blood circulation, 41
blood flow, 42, 48
blood pressure, 57, 61, 150
blood smear, 68, 167
blood supply, 110
blood transfusion, 40, 47, 53, 54, 85, 96, 108, 121, 136, 137, 138, 140
blood transfusions, 40, 47, 136, 137, 138
bloodstream, 26, 129
body weight, 4, 47, 124
bone, vii, viii, ix, 3, 35, 36, 37, 38, 39, 40, 41, 42, 43, 44, 45, 46, 47, 48, 50, 51, 57, 58, 63, 66, 67, 85, 90, 100, 101, 112, 129, 134, 137, 155, 158, 159
bone biology, 44
bone cells, 41
bone form, ix, 36, 41, 43, 45, 46
bone growth, 40
bone marrow, ix, 3, 38, 40, 42, 46, 50, 51, 58, 63, 66, 67, 90, 100, 101, 129, 134, 137, 155, 158, 159
bone marrow transplant, ix, 50
bone mass, viii, 36, 38, 39, 40, 41, 42, 45, 46, 47
bone mineral content, 46
bone resorption, ix, 36, 37, 38, 39, 43, 44, 45, 46, 47
bones, 40, 51
brain, ix, 7, 27, 28, 32, 49, 112
Brazil, 49, 53
breast cancer, 118
breathlessness, 110
budding, 68

C

cachexia, 4
calcium, 30, 45, 47, 56, 58, 62
cancer, xi, 96, 99, 107, 110, 117, 118, 119, 120, 121
capillary, 112
carbohydrate, 138
cardiac arrhythmia, 150
cardiac operations, 121
cardiac output, vii, 1, 6, 104, 105
cardiac reserve, 6
cardiac surgery, 17, 113
cardiogenic shock, 4
cardiomyopathy, 7, 160
cardiorespiratory disease, 104
cardiovascular disease, x, xi, xii, 6, 10, 66, 79, 87, 104, 118, 123, 139, 142, 147, 148
cardiovascular risk, 151, 162
caregivers, 53
catecholamines, 39
category a, 69
catheter, 153
causal relationship, 7
CD8+, 83
cell culture, 25
cell cycle, 73
cell line(s), 67, 68, 69, 87
cerebral cortex, 113
chelates, 21, 22
chemical, 22
chemical properties, 22
chemotherapeutic agent, 67
chemotherapy, x, 58, 67, 81, 86, 88, 94, 118, 136
Chicago, 133

Index

children, xi, 21, 29, 30, 33, 53, 54, 56, 58, 61, 62, 63, 99, 101, 124, 127, 141
Chile, 143
China, 165
chromatography, 75
chromosome, 23, 32, 91, 95
chronic anemia, vii
chronic heart failure, 7, 12, 14, 15, 16, 116, 122, 131, 142, 149
chronic hypoxia, 43
chronic illness, ix, 49, 50, 87
chronic kidney failure, 146, 163
chronic obstructive pulmonary disease (COPD), 40, 46, 111
chronic renal failure, 51, 160
cigarette smoking, 110
circadian rhythm, 127
circulation, 41, 155, 158
citrulline, 62
CKD, xii, 11, 124, 127, 129, 130, 131, 133, 134, 135, 136, 137, 138, 139, 140, 141, 142, 147, 149, 150, 151, 152, 156, 157, 161, 163
classification, 69, 71, 76, 79, 82, 88, 89, 93, 94
cleavage, 43
clinical assessment, 109
clinical problems, 81
clinical symptoms, 51
clinical trials, 59, 85, 101, 120
clone, 72, 76, 91
clusters, 68
coding, 72
coenzyme, 29
cognitive capacities, 81
cognitive development, 124
cognitive function, 141
cognitive impairment, 14, 131
collagen, viii, 36, 39, 41, 42, 43
colorectal cancer, 118
communities, 117
community, 117, 118, 119, 131, 133
comorbidity, 79, 93, 151
complete blood count, 124
compliance, 134

complications, ix, x, xi, 49, 53, 54, 58, 66, 69, 76, 80, 81, 99, 101, 102, 113, 131, 140, 148, 150, 156
compounds, 20, 26, 157
congestive heart failure, 11, 13, 142, 149
consensus, xi, 86, 89, 99, 100, 101, 131, 142
constipation, 134
constituents, 75
consumption, 6, 31, 39, 106
control group, 39
controlled trials, xii, 102, 103, 141, 147, 148
controversial, 9, 10, 11, 12
controversies, 33, 89
convergence, 16
copper, 21, 24, 25, 33, 47, 163
coronary angioplasty, 10
coronary artery disease, 2, 6, 11, 17, 163
coronary heart disease, 116, 118
correlation(s), 23, 24, 41, 47, 104, 107, 109, 110, 111, 113, 117
cortical bone, viii, 36, 39, 40, 45
cortisol, ix, 36, 39, 45
cost, 134, 140
covering, 108
Cox regression, 151
creatinine, 117, 133, 141, 151
CRF, 156
crises, ix, 49, 54, 57, 59
CRP, 127
crystals, 39
CSA, 88
CSF, 82, 83, 94
CT, 117, 148
Cuba, ix, 49, 51
cure, ix, 50, 58, 60, 61
CVD, xii, 131, 147
cyclosporine, 83
cysteine, 26
cytochrome(s), 21, 25, 40
cytogenetics, 68
cytokines, vii, 1, 3, 36, 38, 44, 59, 71, 72, 118
cytometry, 17, 68
cytotoxicity, 90

D

daily living, 111, 114
damages, 27
database, 88, 94, 104
death rate, 58
deaths, 104, 149
decomposition, 29, 31
defecation, 166
defects, 71, 72, 75
defence, 23, 28, 31, 32
deficiencies, 9, 55, 133
deficit, vii, 1
degradation, viii, 24, 36, 44, 75, 129, 139, 155, 163
dehydration, 50, 61
demographic factors, 58
deposits, 54, 74
depression, 110, 122
deprivation, 117
deregulation, 91
derivatives, 21, 95
detection, 53, 163, 166, 167
detoxification, 29
developed countries, 125
developing countries, 7
diabetes, xi, 42, 104, 118, 123, 125, 130, 136, 140, 142, 151
diabetic patients, 104
dialysis, xii, 16, 23, 116, 117, 129, 130, 135, 136, 137, 142, 144, 145, 146, 148, 150, 151, 152, 153, 156, 157, 159, 161, 162, 163, 164
diet, 21, 26, 27, 28, 39, 55, 60, 156
disability, 100, 125
discomfort, 134
disease progression, 91
diseases, vii, viii, 1, 6, 36, 40, 41, 87, 109, 125, 126, 129, 141, 142, 144, 146, 168
disorder, 50
distribution, 27, 42, 51, 52, 68, 74, 126, 155
divergence, 16
diversity, 72
dizziness, 2

DNA, 20, 21, 22, 23, 24, 25, 27, 28, 30, 31, 32, 33, 52, 53, 86, 96
DNA damage, 23, 24, 27, 28, 30, 31, 32, 33
DNA repair, 23, 25
DNA strand breaks, 33
donors, 72
dosing, 120
double-blind trial, 16, 139
DPO, xii, 148, 150, 151, 152, 158, 159
draft, 88
drainage, 105
drugs, ix, 50, 59, 81, 82
duodenum, 25, 74
dysplasia, 67, 68, 69, 71, 73
dyspnea, 2

E

East Asia, 126
egg, 166, 167
eicosapentaenoic acid, 61
elderly population, 140
electron, 20, 24, 25, 74
electron microscopy, 74
electrons, 21
electrophoresis, 75
ELISA, 91
endothelial cells, 28, 31, 44
endothelial dysfunction, 139, 162
endothelium, 50, 51
end-stage renal disease, 130, 148, 160
energy, 47, 55, 60, 110
energy expenditure, 55, 60
England, 31
environment(s), 43, 112
enzymatic activity, 27, 43
enzyme(s), viii, 20, 22, 24, 25, 28, 29, 30, 40, 41, 43, 44, 74, 131, 139
EPA, 57
epidemiologic, viii, 35, 38
epigenetic alterations, 86
epithelial cells, 155, 156
erythrocytes, 21, 28, 31, 51, 57, 61, 63, 75, 92
erythroid cells, 69, 155

erythropoietin, vii, xi, xii, 1, 3, 7, 11, 12, 13, 74, 82, 89, 94, 99, 103, 105, 114, 119, 122, 129, 131, 134, 136, 147, 148, 151, 160, 164
ESRD, 148, 150, 157, 162
estrogen, 38, 42
ethnicity, 124
etiology, 2, 11, 142
Europe, 126, 152, 154, 161
evidence, viii, x, xi, xii, 11, 35, 38, 55, 58, 68, 75, 89, 99, 100, 101, 102, 105, 109, 113, 140, 142, 147, 151, 158, 159, 163
evolution, ix, x, 7, 66, 67, 69, 72, 76, 77, 78, 79, 87, 88, 93, 95
exclusion, 76
excretion, 26, 56, 155
exercise, 7, 16, 38, 39, 111, 112, 119, 121, 122, 139
exercise performance, 111, 112, 122
exertion, 113
exposure, 23, 57, 67, 167
external validation, 107
extraction, 10, 105
extracts, 105

F

failure to thrive, 101
fasting, 56, 128
fat, 42, 44
fatty acids, 55
FDA, 59, 153
Fe deficiency anaemia, viii, ix, 20, 22, 28, 29, 36, 40, 42, 45
femur, ix, 36, 39, 45
ferritin, xii, 8, 26, 27, 30, 73, 84, 85, 86, 127, 128, 130, 134, 138, 148, 153, 154, 155, 156, 157, 158, 162, 163
ferrous ion, 22
fever, 53
fibers, 43
fibrinolytic, 4
fibromyalgia, 111
fibrosis, 68
filtration, 129, 130, 148

fish, 167, 169
fistulas, 152
flexibility, 39, 100
fluid, 11, 58, 108
folate, x, 55, 56, 63, 66, 70, 166
folic acid, ix, 9, 49, 55
food, 135
Ford, 145
formation, viii, ix, 11, 19, 20, 22, 36, 37, 41, 43, 45, 72, 74
fractures, viii, 36, 40, 46, 47, 48, 58
fragility, 57, 58, 61
France, 1, 152, 153
free radicals, 25, 31, 57
fruits, 55
functional capacity, vii, 1, 10, 111
fusion, 37

G

gallstones, 51
gastric mucosa, 143
gastrin, 127
gastritis, 127
gastrocnemius, 113
gastrointestinal bleeding, xi, 115, 123
gastrointestinal tract, 129, 134
gene expression, 43, 76
gene mapping, 91
gene promoter, 86
gene therapy, ix, 50, 58, 60
gene transfer, 63
genes, 37, 44, 72, 73, 75, 86, 91
genetic alteration, 75
genetics, 68
genomics, 52, 64
Germany, 152
gestation, 128
glomerulus, 156
glucocorticoids, 39
glucose, 55, 126
glutamic acid, 50
glutathione, 24, 26, 31
glycerol, 106
glycine, 134

goat milk, 31
Greece, ix, 49
growth, 21, 36, 38, 40, 48, 51, 55, 94, 101
growth factor, 36, 94
guidance, 86, 101, 102, 113, 127
guidelines, xi, 10, 94, 99, 100, 101, 102, 105, 108, 110, 113, 114, 115, 121, 136, 145, 158, 160, 161

H

H. pylori, 127
haemopoiesis, 101
hair, 40
half-life, 82
harmful effects, 156, 159
health, 7, 62, 63, 104, 108, 120, 139, 141, 150
health status, 7
heart conditions, vii, 1
heart disease, vii, 1, 2, 4, 6, 10, 12, 17, 54, 59, 115, 121
heart failure, 2, 3, 4, 5, 6, 7, 8, 9, 10, 11, 12, 14, 16, 102, 116, 118, 131, 139, 142, 146, 150, 159
heart rate, 6
height, 55
Helicobacter pylori, 127
hematocrit, 10, 16, 117, 118, 148
hematology, ix, 66, 67, 143, 145
hematopoietic stem cells, ix, 66, 67
heme, 25, 33, 74, 135, 144, 155
hemochromatosis, 41, 46, 157
hemodialysis, 16, 40, 48, 144, 145, 146, 152, 160, 161, 162, 163, 164
hemoglobin, vii, viii, x, xii, 1, 2, 8, 9, 10, 11, 12, 15, 23, 31, 36, 39, 40, 42, 45, 46, 50, 51, 52, 53, 54, 57, 59, 62, 63, 66, 71, 75, 76, 79, 80, 81, 82, 87, 116, 117, 121, 141, 143, 147, 148, 155, 160, 161, 166
hemoglobinopathies, 50, 62, 127
hemolytic anemia, 56
hemorrhage, 4, 21
hepatocytes, 28, 129
heterogeneity, 76, 103

HFP, 14
histone, 33
HLA, 58, 83
homeostasis, 15, 24, 26, 42, 56, 74, 75, 129, 162
homocysteine, 56, 63
Hong Kong, 142
hookworm, 126, 166, 167, 168
hormone(s), 36, 38, 129
hospital death, 10
hospitalization, 7, 116, 131, 149, 150, 156
host, 58, 67, 155
HSCT, 58, 81, 85, 86, 88
human body, 85, 155
Hunter, 120
hybrid, 59
hydrogen peroxide, 25, 28, 29, 31
hydroxide, 135
hydroxyapatite, 39
hydroxyl, 20, 24, 25, 31
hypermethylation, 71
hyperplasia, 40, 51
hypersensitivity, 136
hypertension, xi, 123, 125, 140
hypertrophy, 6, 148, 161
hypothesis, 39, 59, 72, 148
hypoxemia, 6, 39
hypoxia, ix, 6, 36, 42, 43, 44, 112, 113, 129, 130, 139, 160
hypoxia-inducible factor, 44, 139

I

ibuprofen, 54
idiopathic, 67
IFNγ, 72
imbalances, 37
immune system, 58
immunity, 53
immunization, 54
immunohistochemistry, 68
immunomodulatory, 81
impairments, 41
improvements, 85, 113, 126
in vitro, 32, 33, 43, 45, 59, 72, 86, 90

in vivo, 43, 59, 86, 89
incidence, ix, 15, 54, 66, 67, 68, 135, 150
independence, 84
India, ix, 49, 51, 52
individuals, ix, 49, 58, 87, 105, 109, 111
induction, 44, 58, 59, 63
infants, 52
infarction, 8, 40
infection, 52, 55, 56, 73, 127, 153, 166, 167, 168, 169
inferiority, 109, 121
inflammation, 8, 11, 15, 42, 44, 57, 73, 86, 127, 128, 129, 130, 131, 133, 139, 142, 153, 155, 157
inflammatory disease, 134
inflammatory responses, 71
infrared spectroscopy, 122
inhibition, 43, 95, 139
inhibitor, 4, 10, 139
initiation, 67, 86, 101, 150, 151, 161
injections, 138
injury, 59, 134, 139, 143, 156, 160, 163
integration, 79, 93
intensive care unit, 115
interferon, 90
internalization, 27, 129, 155, 163
intervention, 10, 17, 53, 81, 87, 110
intestine, 26, 155, 166
intoxication, 30
intramuscular injection, 56
ions, 21
iron deficiency anemia, vii, 7, 21, 30, 31, 32, 33, 141, 144, 145, 166
iron transport, 129, 155
iron utility, vii, xii, 148, 153, 154
irradiation, 23
ISC, 51
ischemia, 8, 44, 51, 151
isolation, 127
Italy, ix, 49, 152, 153

J

Japan, xii, 147, 148, 151, 152, 153, 154, 158, 159, 161

K

karyotype, 68, 81, 82, 86
kidney(s), vii, xi, xii, 1, 4, 9, 11, 16, 17, 25, 44, 51, 103, 105, 117, 123, 124, 129, 130, 136, 141, 142, 144, 145, 146, 147, 148, 152, 156, 160, 161, 163
kinetics, 55

L

laboratory tests, 8, 127
lactate dehydrogenase, 9, 84
L-arginine, 57
Latin America, 126
lead, xi, 3, 6, 7, 22, 25, 39, 51, 99, 105, 114, 125, 134
leakage, 6
lesions, 14, 42, 156
leukemia, 69, 74, 90, 96
leukocytes, 25
liberation, 28
life expectancy, xii, 59, 79, 86, 92, 101, 148
ligand, 10, 37
light, 17, 74, 112, 157, 169
light transmission, 17
lipid metabolism, 55, 56
lipid peroxidation, viii, 20, 22, 24, 25, 27, 28, 29, 31, 32
lipids, 20, 25, 27
liquid chromatography, 53
liver, 5, 24, 25, 26, 27, 28, 30, 44, 54, 79, 86, 127, 154, 155
liver cells, 5, 30
liver cirrhosis, 54
liver disease, 86, 127
localization, 68
longitudinal study, 117, 118
loss of appetite, 110
low risk, 85
lower lip, 27
lumen, 27, 135
lung cancer, 117
Luo, 90

lymphocytes, 23, 27, 32, 72
lysine, 43, 59

M

macromolecules, 21
macrophages, 41, 74, 129, 156
magnesium, 30, 45, 57, 61, 62
major depression, 59
malabsorption, 124
malaria, 52, 100, 127, 167, 168
malignancy, 107, 127, 133
management, vii, ix, xi, xiii, 50, 53, 54, 55, 60, 62, 88, 95, 96, 100, 109, 115, 119, 124, 128, 138, 140, 141, 142, 143, 145, 152, 153, 161, 164, 165, 166
manganese, 24
marrow, 15, 46, 67, 71, 74, 90, 129, 137, 159
mass, 36, 37, 39, 40, 42, 43, 74, 104, 105, 106, 117, 118, 152, 160
matrix, viii, ix, 36, 38, 41, 42, 43, 45, 74
measurement(s), 105, 111, 112, 113, 119, 124, 127, 130, 134
median, x, 58, 66, 67, 70, 75, 76, 78, 80, 81, 82, 84, 86, 136
medical, 50, 51, 54, 102, 103, 113, 114, 142, 143
Medicare, 162
medication, 54, 59, 143
medicine, 61, 142, 143, 144, 145, 146
Mediterranean countries, ix, 49, 51
mellitus, 130, 136, 140, 142
meningitis, 54
mental fatigue, 108
meta-analysis, 12, 16, 116
metabolic, 61
metabolic intermediates, 26
metabolic pathways, 23
metabolism, vii, 4, 13, 26, 31, 33, 38, 39, 40, 41, 45, 46, 56, 91, 105, 159, 162, 163, 164
metabolites, 23, 33
metal ion(s), 21
metals, 21

methylation, 86, 96
MFI, 108, 109
mice, 59, 60
micronutrients, 55, 56
microscopy, 74
Middle East, 126
mineral bone content, viii, 35, 38, 45
mineral bone density, viii, 35, 38
mineralization, viii, 36, 37, 39, 40, 41, 45, 47
mitochondria, 25, 32, 74, 75, 92
mitochondrial damage, 75
mitochondrial DNA, 32
mitral stenosis, 6
mitral valve, 13
models, 24, 39, 42
modifications, 42
molecular oxygen, 43
molecules, 22, 142
morbidity, x, 8, 40, 53, 54, 60, 66, 79, 80, 87, 104, 116, 124, 156, 160
morphology, 47, 68, 160
mortality, xii, 4, 6, 7, 8, 9, 10, 11, 12, 13, 15, 17, 53, 54, 59, 60, 80, 85, 101, 102, 103, 104, 116, 117, 118, 131, 140, 143, 147, 148, 152, 153, 154, 156, 158, 160, 161
mortality rate, 152, 153, 156, 158
Moses, 15
motivation, 108
MRI, 121, 154, 157, 162
mRNA, 158
mtDNA, 25
mucosa, 5, 27
multidimensional, 81
multiple myeloma, 117
multipotent, 71
multivariate analysis, 7, 92, 117, 118
murmur, 2
muscles, 26, 155
mutation(s), 32, 50, 52, 71, 73, 74, 75, 85, 91, 92
myelodysplasia, xi, 92, 95, 99, 107, 113, 133

Index

myelodysplastic syndromes, vii, 89, 90, 91, 92, 93, 94, 95, 96, 97, 107, 110, 119, 120
myeloid cells, 82
myeloproliferative disorders, 89
myocardial infarction, 8, 13, 15, 149, 150, 163
myocardial ischemia, 6, 10, 11, 12
myocardial necrosis, 8
myocardium, 6
myoglobin, 155

N

National Health and Nutrition Examination Survey (NHANES), 125, 130, 131, 133
nausea, 134
necrosis, 110
negative outcomes, 131
nematode, 166
neonates, 113
neoplasm, 69, 76
nephrologist, 152
nephron, 156
neurodegenerative diseases, 31
neurological disease, 31
neurotoxicity, 84
neutropenia, 81, 84
neutrophils, 57, 60, 68, 71
New England, 115, 117, 142, 144, 145, 146
New Zealand, 122, 152
nitric oxide, 10, 20, 50, 57, 167, 168
normal development, 124
North Africa, 126
North America, 126
NSAIDs, 54
nuclei, 68
nucleus, 68
nursing home, 131, 143
nutrient(s), 54, 55, 28, 38, 60, 133
nutrition, xi, 123, 141, 144
nutritional deficiencies, 37, 166
nutritional status, 56

O

obstruction, 6, 51
Oceania, 143
omega-3, 55, 57
opioids, 54
organ(s), x, 14, 26, 28, 51, 54, 55, 66, 74, 80, 87, 112, 131
organelles, 75
organism, 21, 22, 28
orthostatic hypotension, 11
osmolality, 138
osmotic stress, 63
ossification, 57
osteoclast activity, ix, 36, 44
osteomyelitis, 40
osteopenia, viii, 35, 38
osteoporosis, viii, 36, 38, 40, 41, 42, 46
oxidation, 21, 28, 30, 31, 33
oxidative damage, viii, 20, 22, 24, 28, 31, 57
oxidative stress, viii, 20, 22, 23, 28, 29, 30, 31, 32, 33, 55, 57, 60, 61, 139, 154, 156
oxygen, vii, ix, 1, 6, 8, 10, 14, 20, 21, 24, 36, 39, 42, 43, 45, 47, 51, 54, 56, 75, 104, 105, 106, 111, 112, 113, 122, 139, 155, 166
oxygen consumption, 6, 106, 111
oxygen delivery, ix, 6, 10, 14, 36, 42, 45, 75, 104, 105, 112, 139

P

p53, 73, 91
Pacific, 126
pain, 2, 40, 51, 54, 119
palliative, 107, 121
parallel, x, 66, 69, 71
parasite(s), xiii, 165, 167
parasitic anemia, vii, xiii, 165, 166
parasitic diseases, 168
parasitic infection, 167
parathyroid hormone, viii, 36
pathogenesis, vii, 1, 2, 54, 59, 91, 92, 163

Index

pathology, 57, 83, 143, 167
pathophysiological, ix, 50, 60, 131
pathophysiology, vii, 1, 2, 50, 71, 162
penicillin, 53
peptide, 5, 7, 129, 136
perfusion, 10, 106, 113
perinatal, 104, 118
peripheral blood, 27, 31, 33, 67, 68, 69
peripheral blood mononuclear cell (PBMC), 23, 31, 33
peripheral vascular disease, 111, 150
pernicious anemia, viii, 36, 40, 46, 169
peroxidation, viii, 20, 22, 25, 27, 29, 30
peroxide, 25
pharmaceutical(s), ix, 50
pharmacokinetics, 143
pharmacology, 162
phenotype, 44, 67
Philadelphia, 92
phosphate, 29, 62, 126
phosphorus, 30, 45
phosphorylation, 33
physical activity, 21, 107
physicians, 108, 120
Physiological, 61
physiology, 38
placebo, 16, 60, 94, 95, 136, 139, 150
placenta, 44, 53
plasma levels, 56
plasma membrane, 26, 155
plasminogen, 4, 10
platelet aggregation, 17, 59
platelet count, 71, 73, 84
platelets, 4, 21, 39, 57, 60, 68, 69
pneumococcus, 51
policy, 121
pollution, 23
polymerization, 50
polymorphism(s), 72, 90
polypeptide, 135, 144
polysaccharide, 54
polyunsaturated fat, 33, 57
polyunsaturated fatty acids, 33
population, ix, xi, 2, 7, 11, 38, 52, 66, 67, 68, 87, 101, 102, 103, 104, 107, 114, 117, 120, 123, 125, 135, 137, 139, 140, 142, 157, 167
population growth, xi, 123
porosity, 40
positive correlation, 74
post-transplant, 58
potential benefits, 139
precursor cells, 72, 90
pregnancy, 5, 104, 118, 124, 128, 141
premature death, 54
prematurity, 53, 124
preparation, 43, 138, 143, 152
preschool children, 124
preservation, 151
prevention, 53, 167
priapism, 51, 54
probability, 82, 83
progenitor cells, 68, 72
proglottid, 167
prognosis, x, 7, 63, 67, 76, 81, 85, 86, 87, 89, 111, 116, 154, 158, 159, 162
pro-inflammatory, 3, 72
proliferation, ix, 36, 37, 43, 67, 71, 72
proline, 42
prophylactic, 53, 55, 59
prophylaxis, 53, 81
prostate cancer, 117
prosthetic device, 11
proteasome, 163
protection, viii, 4, 20, 22, 23, 29, 32, 57, 151
protective role, 31
proteins, 20, 21, 27, 28, 30, 71
proteinuria, 131
public health, xii, 165, 166
pulmonary edema, 2
pulmonary hypertension, 101, 111

Q

quality of life, x, xi, xii, 7, 60, 66, 81, 82, 85, 88, 94, 99, 101, 102, 103, 106, 107, 108, 109, 110, 114, 116, 117, 119, 120, 139, 147, 148
Queensland, 123

Index

R

race, 106, 119
radiation therapy, 67
radicals, 20, 21, 24, 25, 155, 156
reactant, 8
reactions, 22, 24, 28, 29, 32, 33, 39, 44, 72, 136, 138
reactive oxygen, 20, 22, 23, 75, 139, 157
reactivity, 138
reagents, 134
receptors, 10, 28, 106, 155
recommendations, 56, 100
recovery, vii, 31, 39
recycling, 56
red blood cell count, 5
red blood cell indices, 75
red blood cells, vii, 1, 5, 23, 26, 28, 32, 33, 56, 59, 63, 159
redistribution, 155
registry, x, 10, 14, 66, 71, 88
regression, 79, 92
regression model, 79, 92
rehabilitation program, 111
relapses, 82
relief, xi, 54, 82, 100
remission, 83
remodelling, 36, 41, 139
renal dysfunction, 3, 131
renal failure, 42, 151, 156, 160
renal osteodystrophy, 41
renal replacement therapy, 149
renin, 3
repair, viii, 13, 20, 22, 23, 25, 31, 32, 36
replication, 23
requirements, 17, 21, 36, 55, 58, 81, 82, 85, 96, 110, 115, 140, 163
residues, 41, 42
resistance, viii, xii, 3, 9, 36, 38, 39, 45, 131, 147
respiration, 44
response, 6, 17, 23, 38, 43, 73, 75, 82, 83, 84, 86, 87, 88, 94, 95, 96, 97, 102, 111, 112, 117, 118, 129, 134, 137, 144, 145, 153, 158

responsiveness, 120
retardation, 101
retinol, 56, 61
retinopathy, 51
RH, 32
rheumatoid arthritis, 120
ribonucleotide reductase, 25
ribosome, 73
risk assessment, x, 66, 76, 93
risk factors, vii, xi, 116, 123, 125
risks, 101, 103, 114, 124, 138, 148, 157, 166, 167
ROS, viii, 19, 20, 22, 23, 27, 28, 29, 75

S

safety, xii, 102, 124, 134, 135, 138, 139, 143, 145, 149, 157, 159
salts, 31, 134, 135
saturation, xii, 22, 46, 112, 113, 122, 128, 130, 148, 153, 156, 163
Saudi Arabia, ix, 49, 51, 52
scavengers, 57
schistosomiasis, 127, 168
sclerosis, 40
secrete, 37, 41
secretion, vii, 1, 43
selenium, 24, 30, 33
sensitivity, 7
sepsis, 102
Serbia, 165
serum, viii, xii, 7, 8, 21, 30, 36, 39, 46, 71, 73, 80, 83, 84, 86, 117, 127, 129, 130, 134, 135, 148, 151, 153, 154, 155, 156, 157, 158, 159, 163, 164
serum erythropoietin, 71
serum ferritin, xii, 8, 22, 73, 80, 86, 127, 129, 130, 135, 148, 153, 154, 156, 157, 158, 159, 163
serum iron level, 158
sex, 68, 79, 80, 125, 128, 151
sex chromosome, 68
shape, 50, 51
shear, 6
shortage, 51, 74

shortness of breath, 69
showing, 11, 107, 111, 149
sibling, 58
sickle cell, vii, x, 40, 50, 52, 53, 54, 56, 57, 59, 60, 61, 62, 63, 99, 100, 113, 115, 127
sickle cell anemia, vii, 50, 53, 61, 62, 63
side effects, 134, 135, 140
sideroblastic anemia, 74
signaling pathway, 44, 71
signs, 86, 102
skeleton, 36
skin, 105, 112
small intestine, 32
socioeconomic background, 124
sodium, 58, 137
solid tumors, 119
solubility, 27
somatic mutations, 76
South America, ix, 49, 51
Spain, 19, 35, 152
speciation, 33
species, 20, 22, 23, 75, 139, 157
spectroscopy, 112, 113
speculation, 106
spleen, 26, 51, 155
spongy bone, 38
Spring, 168
sprue, 7
SSA, 126
stability, 10, 22, 25, 31
stabilization, 44
state(s), 3, 4, 10, 21, 28, 33, 36, 38, 42, 50, 56, 71, 72, 101, 106, 111, 120, 124, 129
stem cells, ix, 58, 66, 71
stenosis, 6, 14
sternum, 26, 39
stimulation, 44
storage, 21, 28, 39, 154
stress, viii, 6, 19, 20, 22, 23, 24, 30, 31, 57, 112, 156
stress test, 112
stress testing, 112
stroke, 6, 10, 51, 54, 101, 117, 136, 149, 150
stroke volume, 6

stromal cells, 71
structure, 37
subarachnoid hemorrhage, 51
subgroups, x, 66, 69, 76
sub-Saharan Africa, 63, 126
substrate(s), 44, 48
sucrose, 135, 137
sulfate, 134, 143, 144
sulphur, 40
supervision, 111, 112
supplementation, xi, 10, 30, 32, 55, 56, 57, 60, 61, 124, 135, 137, 139, 141, 144, 162, 166
suppression, 72, 83, 90, 158, 159, 164
surveillance, 72, 124
survival, vii, x, 1, 7, 10, 11, 66, 67, 73, 76, 77, 78, 80, 81, 82, 84, 85, 86, 87, 88, 92, 93, 94, 95, 96, 97, 103, 108, 115, 116, 117, 118, 129, 139, 151, 158
survival rate, 86, 151, 158
susceptibility, viii, 20, 22, 24, 29, 33, 56, 63, 67
Sweden, 152, 153
symbiosis, 13
sympathetic nervous system, 3
symptoms, xi, 2, 4, 10, 11, 55, 57, 82, 85, 100, 102, 105, 107, 108, 109, 110, 114, 119, 120, 131, 138
syndrome, xi, 4, 6, 8, 13, 14, 54, 55, 59, 69, 70, 73, 74, 84, 89, 90, 91, 92, 93, 95, 96, 102, 107, 108, 110, 120, 121, 124, 131, 133, 136, 140
synergistic effect, 82
synthesis, 24, 25, 26, 41, 55, 59, 74, 75, 155

T

T cell, 72
T lymphocytes, 83
tachycardia, 2, 11
tapeworm, 167, 169
target, xii, 11, 63, 84, 110, 113, 139, 147, 149, 151, 153, 158, 160, 161
target population(s), 160

tartrate-resistant acid phosphatase, viii, 36, 41
T-cell receptor, 72, 95
TCR, 72
techniques, ix, 50, 53
tensile strength, 43
tension, 44, 47
testing, 108, 109, 111, 112, 122, 129
Thailand, 165
thalassemia, 40, 46, 47, 62, 75, 76, 89, 92, 115, 127, 133
therapeutic interventions, 37
therapy, xii, 4, 11, 29, 41, 53, 54, 58, 59, 60, 62, 81, 82, 84, 85, 86, 91, 93, 95, 96, 100, 101, 107, 108, 110, 113, 114, 117, 118, 124, 135, 137, 138, 140, 145, 148, 150, 151, 157, 160, 168
thrombocytopenia, 69, 81, 84, 87, 90
thrombus, 6, 11, 13
time periods, 126
tissue, 6, 10, 21, 28, 36, 56, 105, 112, 113, 157
total iron binding capacity, 128
toxic effect, 59
toxicity, 27, 84, 156
toxin, 41
TP53, 73, 85, 91
trafficking, 26, 27, 28, 32, 155
transcription, 43, 44, 72, 90, 139
transcription factors, 43
transferrin, xii, 8, 22, 24, 26, 27, 28, 91, 128, 129, 130, 134, 143, 148, 153, 156, 163
transformation, x, 26, 66, 69, 73, 75, 76, 86
transient ischemic attack, 150
transition metal ions, 21, 163
transplant, 86
transplantation, ix, x, 50, 58, 60, 67, 81, 93, 110, 121, 137, 144, 145, 146, 151
transport, 24, 25, 27, 56, 57, 112
transportation, 166
trauma, 113
trial, 9, 13, 15, 16, 17, 60, 84, 85, 87, 96, 102, 115, 116, 118, 121, 135, 136, 138, 139, 140, 144, 145, 149, 150, 160

triggers, 114
trisomy, 68
tumo(u)r(s), 3, 42, 44, 47, 73, 79, 89, 90
tumor necrosis factor (TNF), 3, 72, 90, 158
Turkey, ix, 49
turnover, 21, 36, 37, 41, 46, 60
type 2 diabetes, 142, 145, 160

U

umbilical cord, 53
United Kingdom (UK), 62, 152
United States (USA), 1, 53, 56, 89, 90, 91, 125, 136, 141, 145, 152, 161
unstable angina, 8
urinalysis, 161
urine, 54, 56, 63

V

vaccine, 167
valine, 50
valve, 6, 9
variables, 21, 73, 76, 83, 129
vascular occlusion, 59
vasodilation, 10
vaso-occlusion, 54
vector, 167
vegetables, 55
velocity, 6, 39
vertebrae, 47
vessels, 51, 106
viscosity, 14, 105, 106
vitamin B1, x, 9, 56, 60, 66, 70, 166
vitamin B12, x, 9, 56, 60, 66, 70, 166
vitamin B12 deficiency, 56
vitamin B6, 56
vitamin C, 38, 55, 57, 61
vitamin D, 36, 38, 40, 46, 57
vitamin D deficiency, 57
vitamin E, 55, 57
vitamins, 55, 56, 57, 60
vomiting, 134

W

walking, 111
water, 58, 131
weakness, 39, 69
well-being, 108
West Africa, 62
World Health Organization (WHO), 2, 50, 51, 52, 53, 54, 55, 64, 69, 70, 71, 79, 82, 89, 93, 94, 124, 127, 134, 141, 143

Y

young women, 141

Z

zinc, 21, 24, 55, 56, 129